CLINICAL CASES in OCULAR ONCOLOGY

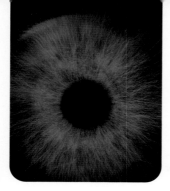

CLINICAL CASES in
OCULAR ONCOLOGY

APARNA RAMASUBRAMANIAN, MD

Director of Retinoblastoma & Ocular Oncology – Children's Wisconsin
Associate Professor of Ophthalmology
Medical College of Wisconsin
Milwaukee, Wisconsin
United States

CAROL L. SHIELDS, MD

Director, Ocular Oncology Service
Wills Eye Hospital
Thomas Jefferson University
Philadelphia, Pennsylvania
United States

ELSEVIER

ELSEVIER
1600 John F. Kennedy Blvd.
Ste 1800
Philadelphia, PA 19103-2899

CLINICAL CASES IN OCULAR ONCOLOGY   ISBN: 978-0-443-12049-7

Notice

Practitioners and researchers must always rely on their own experience and knowledge in evaluating and using any information, methods, compounds or experiments described herein. Because of rapid advances in the medical sciences, in particular, independent verification of diagnoses and drug dosages should be made. To the fullest extent of the law, no responsibility is assumed by Elsevier, authors, editors or contributors for any injury and/or damage to persons or property as a matter of products liability, negligence or otherwise, or from any use or operation of any methods, products, instructions, or ideas contained in the material herein.

Executive Content Strategist: Kayla Wolfe
Senior Content Development Specialist: Vasowati Shome
Content Development Manager: Ranjana Sharma
Publishing Services Manager: Deepthi Unni
Project Manager: Haritha Dharmarajan
Design Direction: Renee Duenow

Working together
to grow libraries in
developing countries

Printed in India
Last digit is the print number: 9 8 7 6 5 4 3 2 1

www.elsevier.com • www.bookaid.org

I dedicate this book to my parents,
my endlessly supportive husband, Raj,
and our loving children, Pranav and Deeksha,
who make everything worthwhile.

On behalf of all the contributing authors,
we dedicate this book to our patients and families
who inspire us to do better every day.

Aparna Ramasubramanian

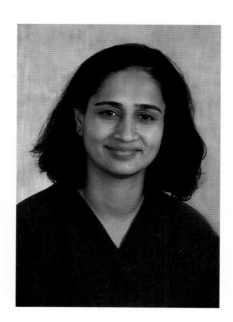

I dedicate this wonderful book
to my husband, Jerry A. Shields, MD,
who spent over 50 years devoted to the field of ocular oncology
while tirelessly working to organize and categorize each eye condition.

I also dedicate this book to our seven children
who have been an everlasting inspiration to us for caring for each patient.

Carol L. Shields

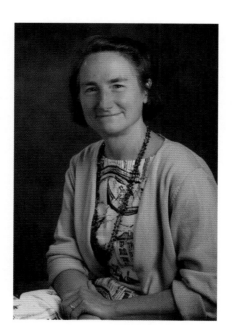

Khushdeep Abhaypal, MBBS, MS
Senior Resident
Department of Ophthalmology
Postgraduate Institute of Medical Education
 & Research
Chandigarh, Punjab
India

Todd Abruzzo, MD
Neurointerventional Radiologist
Radiology
Phoenix Children's Hospital
Phoenix, Arizona
United States

Janelle Marie Fassbender Adeniran, MD, PhD
Vitreoretinal Surgery
Ophthalmology
Bennett & Bloom Eye Centers
Louisville, Kentucky
United States

Kushal Umeshbhai Agrawal, MS Ophthalmology
Fellowship in Ocular Oncology, Fellowship
 in Surgical Retina and Uveitis
Department of Ocular Oncology, Uveitis,
 and Retina
Jupiter Hospital
Ocular Oncology, Uveitis and Retina
Jupiter Hospital
Thane, Maharashtra
India;
Wills Eye Hospital
Ocular Oncology
Wills Eye Hospital
Philadelphia, Pennsylvania
United States

Aneesha Ahluwalia, MD
Resident
Department of Ophthalmology
Stanford University
Palo Alto, California
United States

Amer F. Alsoudi, BS, MD
Department of Ophthalmology
Baylor College of Medicine
Houston, Texas
United States

Rawan Althaqib, MD
Consultant, Assistant Professor
Oculoplastic and Orbit
King Khaled Eye Specialist Hospital
Riyadh, Saudi Arabia

Mattan Arazi, MD
Medical Resident
Department of Ophthalmology
Sheba Medical Center
Ramat Gan, Israel

Komal Bakal, MBBS, DNB Ophthalmology
Fellow, Ophtahlmic Plastic Reconstructive
 Surgery and Ocular Oncology Services
LV Prasad Eye Institute
Kallam Anji Reddy Campus
Hyderabad, Telangana
India

Saaquib Bakhsh, MD
Ophthalmologist
Department of Ophthalmology
Indiana University
School of Medicine
Indianapolis, Indiana
United States

Zeynep Bas, MD
Fellow
Department of Ocular Oncology
Wills Eye Hospital
Philadelphia, Pennsylvania
United States

Jesse L. Berry, MD
Associate Professor of Ophthalmology
Director, Ocular Oncology
Clinical Scholar
Department of Ophthalmology
Children's Hospital Los Angeles
USC Roski Eye Institute
Los Angeles, California
United States

John Bladen, MBBS, BSc, MRCS, PGCert, PhD, FRCOphth
Consultant Ophthalmologist and
    Oculoplastic Surgeon
Kings College Hospital NHS Foundation Trust
London, England
United Kingdom

Elizabeth Miller Bolton, MD
Resident Physician
Department of Ophthalmology
Northwestern University
Chicago, Illinois
United States

Emmanuel Lee Boniao, MD, DPBO
Ophthalmologist
Department of Ophthalmology
Amai Pakpak Medical Center
Marawi City, Philippines;
Department of Ophthalmology
Iligan Polymedic
Iligan City, Philippines

Anderson Brock, BS, COMT, CME
Department of Ocular Oncology
Tennessee Retina
Nashville, Tennessee
United States

Alex H. Brown, BS
Medical Student
University of Arizona College of
    Medicine–Phoenix
Phoenix, Arizona
United States

Sarah Brumley, BS
Summer Intern
Cancer Prevention Research Training Program
University of Texas MD Anderson Cancer
    Center
Houston, Texas
United States;
Research Assistant
Ophthalmology and Vision Sciences
University of Iowa
Iowa City, Iowa
United States

Tommy Bui, BS
Medical Student
Medical College of Georgia
Augusta University
Augusta, Georgia
United States

Mona Camacci, MD, MS
Ophthalmologist
Department of Ophthalmology
Retina Consultants of Charleston
Charleston, South Carolina
United States

Nathalie Cassoux, MD, PhD
Director
Department of Ocular Oncology
Institut Curie
Paris, France

Linda A. Cernichiaro-Espinosa, MD
Postdoctoral Scholar
Department of Ophthalmology
University of Tennessee
Memphis, Tennessee
United States

Chaow Charoenkijkajorn, MD
Assistant Professor
Department of Ophthalmology
University of Arkansas for Medical Science
Little Rock, Arkansas
United States

Bhavna Chawla, MS (Ophthalmology)
Ocular Oncology Service
Dr. Rajendra Prasad Centre for Ophthalmic
    Sciences
All India Institute of Medical Sciences
New Delhi, India

Elliot Cherkas, MD
Ophthalmology Resident
Department of Ophthalmology
Casey Eye Institute
Portland, Oregon
United States

Jared Ching, MB ChB, MPharm, PhD, FRCOphth
Honorary Research Fellow
Ocular Oncology Service
Moorfields Eye Hospital
London, England
United Kingdom

Ratima Chokchaitanasin, MD
Retinal Specialist
Department of Ophthalmology
Ramathibodi Hospital
Bangkok, Thailand

Christopher Compton, MD
Associate Professor
Department of Ophthalmology
University of Louisville
Louisville, Kentucky
United States

Mary Connolly-Wilson, BN, MEd
Genetic Counsellor (retired)
Medical Genetics Program
Eastern Health
St. Johns, Newfoundland and Labrador
Canada

Rachel Curtis, MD, FRCSC
Assistant Professor
Department of Ophthalmology
Queen's University
Kingston, Ontario
Canada

Thomas A. DeCesare, BS
Medical Student
School of Medicine
Creighton University School of Medicine
Phoenix, Arizona
United States

Joseph DeSimone, BS
Medical Student
Department of Ophthalmology
Sidney Kimmel Medical College at Thomas
  Jefferson University
Philadelphia, Pennsylvania
United States;
Medical Student
Department of Ocular Oncology
Wills Eye Hospital
Philadelphia, Pennsylvania
United States

Maura Di Nicola, MD
Assistant Professor
Department of Ophthalmology
Bascom Palmer Eye Institute
Miami, Florida
United States

Helen Dimaras, PhD
Scientist
Department of Ophthalmology and Vision
  Sciences
Hospital for Sick Children
Toronto, Ontario
Canada;
Associate Professor
Department of Ophthalmology and Vision
  Sciences
University of Toronto
Toronto, Ontario
Canada

Philip W. Dockery, MD, MPH
Physician
Jones Eye Institute
University of Arkansas for Medical
  Sciences
Little Rock, Arkansas
United States

S. Elizabeth Dugan, MD
Resident Physician
Ophthalmology and Visual Sciences
University of Louisville
Louisville, Kentucky
United States

Elizabeth Dupuy, MD
Staff Physician
Department of Dermatology
Phoenix Children's Hospital
Phoenix, Arizona
United States

Maya Eiger-Moscovich, MD
Ocular Oncologist and Ophthalmic
  Pathologist
Department of Ophthalmology
Hadassah Medical Center
Jerusalem, Israel

Bita Esmaeli, MD, MA
Professor of Ophthalmology and Plastic
    Surgery
Orbital Oncology & Ophthalmic Plastic
    Surgery Service
Department of Plastic Surgery
MD Anderson Cancer Center
Houston, Texas
United States

Ido Didi Fabian, MD
Consultant Ocular Oncologist
Department of Ophthalmology
Sheba Medical Center
Ramat Gan, Israel

Roxana Fu, MD
Associate Professor
Department of Ophthalmology
University of Pittsburgh
Pittsburgh, Pennsylvania
United States

Anat Galor, MD, MSPH
Professor
Department of Ophthalmology
Bascom Palmer Eye Institute
University of Miami
Miami, Florida
United States;
Staff Physician
Miami VAMC
Miami, Florida
United States

Kusumitha B. Ganesh, MBBS, MD
Senior Resident
Department of Ophthalmology
Dr. Rajendra Prasad Centre for Ophthalmic
    Sciences
All India Institute of Medical Sciences
New Delhi, India

Bria George, PharmD
Medical Student
College of Medicine
Florida International University
Miami, Florida
United States

Fariba Ghassemi, MD
Professor
Department of Ophthalmology
Tehran University of Medical Sciences
Farabi Hospital, Tehran
Iran, Islamic Republic of Iran

Dan S. Gombos, MD FACS
Professor & Chief, Section of Ophthalmology
Department of Head and Neck Surgery
MD Anderson Cancer Center
Houston, Texas
United States

Alejandra Etulain González, MD
Alejandra Etulain
Pediatric Opthalmologic
Hospital Infantil Teletón de Oncología,
    Queretaro
Queretaro, Mexico

Efren Gonzalez, MD
Director, Ocular Oncology Center
Department of Ophthalmology
Boston Children's Hospital
Boston, Massachusetts
United States

Eric D. Hansen, MD
Assistant Professor of Ophthalmology
Director of Ocular Oncology
Department of Ophthalmology and
    Visual Sciences
John A Moran Eye Center
Salt Lake City, Utah
United States

Lindsey Hoffman, DO, MS
Staff Physician
Center for Cancer and Blood Disorders
Phoenix Children's Hospital
Phoenix, Arizona
United States

Sang H. Hong, MD
Assistant Professor
Department of Ophthalmology and Visual
    Sciences
Medical College of Wisconsin
Milwaukee, Wisconsin
United States

Jaxon Huang, BHSc
Research Fellow
Department of Ophthalmology
University of Miami
Miami, Florida
United States

Saumya Jakati, MD
Pathologist
Ophthalmic Pathology Laboratory
LV Prasad Eye Institute
Hyderabad, Telangana
India

Abigail Jebaraj, MD
Ophthalmologist
Department of Ophthalmology
Moran Eye Center
University of Utah
Salt Lake City, Utah
United States

Jocelyn Juarez, MD
Pediatric Oncologist
Hospital Infantil De Oncologia "HITO"
Querétaro, Qro.
Mexico

Denis Jusufbegovic, MD
Department of Ophthalmology
Indiana University School of Medicine
Indianapolis, Indiana
United States

Nicholas E. Kalafatis, MD
Resident
Department of Ophthalmology
Indiana University School of Medicine
Indianapolis, Indiana
United States

Swathi Kaliki, MD
Head of Department
Ocular Oncology
LV Prasad Eye Institute
Hyderabad, Telangana
India

Junne Kamihara, MD, PhD
Physician
Department of Pediatric Oncology
Dana-Farber Cancer Institute
Boston, Massachusetts
United States

Carol Karp, MD
Professor of Ophthalmology
Bascom Palmer Eye Institute
University of Miami Miller School of Medicine
Miami, Florida
United States

Caitlin Kelley-Smith, BS
Medical Student (MS4)
School of Medicine
Creighton University
Phoenix, Arizona
United States

Brandon Kennedy, MD
Ophthalmology Resident
Department of Ophthalmology
Moran Eye Center
University of Utah
Salt Lake City, Utah
United States

Farid Khan, MD
Ophthalmologist
Department of Surgery
Omaha Veterans Affairs Medical Center
Omaha, Nebraska
United States

Vikas Khetan, MD, FRCS, FRCO, FRCS(Ed)
Professor
Department of Ophthalmology
Flaum Eye institute
Rochester, New York
United States

Emine Kilic, MD
Associate Professor
Ophthalmologist, Ocular Oncology and
    Vitreoretinal Surgery
Department of Ophthalmology
Erasmus Medical Center
Rotterdam, Netherlands

Gulunay Kiray, MD, FEBO, MRCSEd
Physician
Retinoblastoma Service
Royal London Hospital, Barts Health Trust
London, United Kingdom

Hila Goldberg Kremer, MD
Orbital Oncology and Ophthalmic Plastic
  Surgery
Department of Plastic Surgery
University of Texas MD Anderson Cancer
  Center
Houston, Texas
United States

Thanaporn Kritfuangfoo, MD
Ophthalmologist
Vajira, Ratchathewi
Thailand

Sara E. Lally, MD
Attending Surgeon
Oncology Service
Wills Eye Hospital
Philadelphia, Pennsylvania
United States

Hart G.W. Lidov, MD, PhD
Neuropathologist
Department of Pathology
Boston Childrens Hospital
Boston, Massachusetts
United States

Andre Litwin, FRCOphth
Consultant Ophthalmic and Oculoplastic
  Surgeon
Queen Victoria Hospital NHS Foundation
  Trust
East Grinstead, West Sussex
England, United Kingdom

Elyana Vittoria Tessa Locatelli, BS
Research Associate
Department of Corneal and External Diseases
Bascom Palmer Eye Institute
Miami, Florida
United States;
Research Associate
Department of Surgical Services
Bruce W. Carter VA Medical Center
Miami, Florida
United States

Christopher Patrick Long, MD
Resident Physician
Department of Ophthalmology
USC Roski Eye Institute
Los Angeles, California
United States

Jocelyn Lugo, MD
Hospital infantil Teletón de oncología,
  Querétaro, México

Hanna Luong, BS
Medical Student
Department of Ophthalmology
Mayo Clinic Alix School of Medicine
Scottsdale, Arizona
United States

Joseph Luvisi, MD
Ophthalmologist
Storm Eye Institute
Medical University of South Carolina
Charleston, South Carolina
United States

Lakshmi Mahesh, MBBS, DNB
Ophthalmologist
Department of Orbit and Oculoplasty
Sakra World Hospital
Bangalore, Karnataka
India

Anthony Mai, MD
Resident
Department of Ophthalmology
Moran Eye Center
University of Utah
Salt Lake City, Utah
United States

Aditya Maitray, MSI
Senior Consultant
Department ot Vitreoretina Services
Aravind Eye Hospital
Chennai, Tamil Nadu
India

Azza M.Y. Maktabi, MD
Consultant
Saudi Board of Ophthalmology
Pathology and Laboratory Medicine
  Department
King Khalid Eye Specialist Hospital
Riyadh, Saudi Arabia

Denis Malaise, MD, MSc
Ophthalmologist
Department of Ocular Oncology
Institut Curie
Paris, France

Raman Malhotra, FRCS
Consultant Ophthalmologist
Queen Victoria Hospital
East Grinstead, West Sussex
London, England
United Kingdom

Azzam Malkawi, BA
Medical Student
Department of Ophthalmology
University of Louisville
Louisville, Kentucky
United States

Ashwin Mallipatna, MD
Head of Retinoblastoma Program
Department of Ophthalmology and Vision
 Sciences
Hospital for Sick Children
Toronto, Ontario
Canada;
Assistant Professor
Department of Ophthalmology and Vision
 Sciences
University of Toronto
Toronto, Ontario
Canada

**Fairooz Puthiyapurayil Manjandavida, MBBS,
MD, FACS**
Director
Department of Oculoplasty, Orbit and
 Ocular Oncology
HORUS Specialty Eye Care
Bengaluru, Karnataka
India

Alexandre Matet, MD, PhD
Deputy Head of Department
Department of Ocular Oncology
Institut Curie
Paris, France;
Associate Professor
Faculty of Medicine
Université Paris Cité
Paris, France

Smitha Menon, MD
Clinical Associate Professor
Division of Hematology and Oncology
University of Washington School of Medicine
Montlake, Washington
United States

Dilip K.R. Mishra , MD
Consultant Pathologist
lV Prasad
Hyderabad, Telangana
India

Alexandre Moulin, MD, PD, MER
Head of Eye Pathology Laboratory
Department of Ophthalmology
Jules-Gonin Eye Hospital
Lausanne, Switzerland

Prithvi Mruthyunjaya, MD, MHS
Professor
Department of Ophthalmology and
 Radiation Oncology
Byers Eye Institute at Stanford University
Palo Alto, California
United States

Kaustubh Mulay, DNB
Consultant Ophthalmic Pathologist
National Reporting Centre for Ophthalmic
 Pathology (NRCOP)
Centre For Sight
Hyderabad, Telangana
India

Guy Simon Negretti, MA, MB BChir, FRCOphth
Consultant Ocular Oncologist
Department of Ocular Oncology
Moorfields Eye Hospital
London, England
United Kingdom;
Consultant Ocular Oncologist
The London Retinoblastoma Service
The Royal London Hospital
London, England
United Kingdom;
Consultant Ophthalmologist
Department of Ophthalmology
Surrey and Sussex Healthcare NHS Trust
Redhill, England
United Kingdom

Sahar Parvizi, BMBCh, MA, FRCOphth
Consultant Ophthalmologist
Department of Ophthalmology
Surrey and Sussex NHS Healthcare Trust
Redhill, England
United Kingdom

Bhupendra C.K. Patel, MD, FRCS, FRCOphth
Professor
Department of Ophthalmology and
    Department of Plastic Surgery
University of Utah
Salt Lake City, Utah
United States

Sarah Beth Pike, BA
Medical Student
Department of Ophthalmology
Keck School of Medicine of USC
Los Angeles, California
United States

Aparna Ramasubramanian, MD
Director of Retinoblastoma & Ocular
    Oncology – Children's Wisconsin
Associate Professor of Ophthalmology
Medical College of Wisconsin
Milwaukee, Wisconsin
United States

Maddy Ashwin Reddy, FRCOphth, MD(Res)
Lead Clinician
Retinoblastoma Unit
Royal London Hospital
Barts Health NHS Trust
London, England
United Kingdom;
Honorary Clinical Senior Lecturer
Queen Mary University of London
London, England
United Kingdom;
Honorary Consultant
Department of Paediatrics
Moorfields Eye Hospital NHS Foundation
    Trust
London, England
United Kingdom

David Reichstein, MD
Department of Vitreoretinal Surgery and
    Ocular Oncology
Tennessee Retina
Nashville, Tennessee
United States

Margaret Reynolds, MD, MSc
Assistant Professor
Department of Ophthalmology
Washington University St. Louis
St. Louis, Missouri
United States

Pukhraj Rishi, MBBS, MS, FRCS, FRCSEd, FACS
Associate Professor
Truhlsen Eye Institute
University of Nebraska Medical Centre
Omaha, Nebraska
United States

Aurora Rodriguez, BS
Medical Student
School of Medicine
Creighton University
Phoenix, Arizona
United States

Duangnate Rojanaporn, MD
Associate Professor
Department of Ophthalmology
Ramathibodi Hospital
Bangkok, Thailand

Christine Ryu, MD
Resident
Ophthalmology
Truhlsen Eye Institute
Omaha, Nebraska
United States

**Mandeep Sagoo, MB, PhD, FRCS (Ed),
FRCOphth**
Professor of Ophthalmology and Ocular
    Oncology
Department of Ocular Oncology
Moorfields Eye Hospital and UCL Institute
    of Ophthalmology
London, England
United Kingdom

Manu Saini, MD
Assistant Professor
Department of Ophthalmology
Advanced Eye Center
Postgraduate Institute of Medical Education
    & Research
Chandigarh, Punjab
India

Emil Anthony Say, MD
Assistant Professor
Storm Eye Institute
Medical University of South Carolina
Charleston, South Carolina
United States

Ann Schalenbourg, MD
Médecin Adjoint
Department of Adult Ocular Oncology
Jules-Gonin Eye Hospital
University of Lausanne
Lausanne, Switzerland

Amy Schefler, MD, FACS, FACRS
Associate Professor of Clinical Ophthalmology
Department of Ophthalmology
Weill Cornell Medicine
Houston, Texas
United States

Mrittika Sen, MD, FICO, MRCSEd
Consultant
Department of Ocular Oncology and
 Oculoplasty Services
Raghunath Netralaya
Mumbai, Maharashtra
India

Carol L. Shields, MD
Director, Ocular Oncology Service
Wills Eye Hospital
Thomas Jefferson University
Philadelphia, Pennsylvania
United States

Usha Singh, MS
Physician
Department of Ophthalmology
Postgraduate Institute of Medical Education
 & Research
Chandigarh, Punjab
India

Kareem Sioufi, MD
Acting Instructor
Department of Ophthalmology
University of Washington
Seattle, Washington
United States

Henry C. Skrehot, BA
Medical Student
School of Medicine
Baylor College of Medicine
Houston, Texas
United States

Andrew Stacey, MD, MS
Associate Professor, Ocular Oncology
Department of Ophthalmology
University of Washington
Seattle, Washington
United States

Christina Stathopoulos, MD
Physician
Department of Ocular Oncology
Jules Gonin Eye Hospital
Lausanne, Switzerland

Gangadhara Sundar, MD, FRCSEd, FAMS
Senior Consultant and Head
Orbit and Oculofacial Surgery
Clinical Associate Professor
Department of Ophthalmology
National University Hospital
National University of Singapore
Singapore

Jonathan Thomas, BS
Medical Student
Texas A&M School of Medicine
Dallas, Texas
United States

Wantanee Dangboon Tsutsumi, MD
Instructor in Ophthalmology
Department of Ophthalmology
Songklanagarind University
Hat Yai, Songkhla
Thailand

Elizabeth L. Turner, BS
Medical Student
Department of Biomedical Sciences
Noorda College of Osteopathic Medicine
Provo, Utah
United States

Sravanthi Vegunta, MD
Assistant Professor
Department of Ophthalmology
University of Utah
Salt Lake City, Utah
United States

Vijitha S. Vempuluru, MD, FICO
Consultant Ophthalmologist
Operation Eyesight Universal Institute for
    Eye Cancer
LV Prasad Eye Institute
Hyderabad, Telangana
India

Vicktoria Vishnevskia-Dai, MD
Director of the Ocular Oncology Service
The Goldschleger Eye Institute
Sheba Medical Center, Tel Aviv University
Ramut Gun, Israel;
Head of the Israeli Ocular Oncology Group
    (IOOG)
Honorary Secretary, International Society of
    Ocular Oncology (ISOO)
Vice President Ocular Oncology Group (OOG)

Judith Warner, MD
Clinical Professor of Ophthalmology and
    Neurology
Department of Ophthalmology and Vision
    Sciences
University of Utah
Salt Lake City, Utah
United States

Ezekiel Weis, MD, MPH
Professor
Ophthalmology
University of Alberta
Edmonton, Canada

Nicole West, MD
Oculoplastics Fellow
Department of Ophthalmology
University of Louisville
Louisville, Kentucky
United States

Basil K. Williams, Jr., MD
Associate Professor
Department of Ophthalmology
Bascom Palmer Eye Institute
Miami, Florida
United States

Ethan Willis, BS
Medical Student
College of Medicine
University of Tennessee Health Science Center
Memphis, Tennessee
United States

Antonio Yaghy, MD
Researcher
Department of Retina
New England Eye Center
Boston, Massachusetts
United States

Marielle P. Young, MD
Associate Professor
Department of Ophthalmology
University of Utah
Salt Lake City, Utah
United States

Janice Lasky Zeid, MD
Attending Physician
Division of Ophthalmology
Ann & Robert H. Lurie Children's Hospital
    of Chicago
Chicago, Illinois
United States;
Associate Professor
Department of Ophthalmology
Northwestern University Feinberg School of
    Medicine
Chicago, Illinois
United States

Matthew M. Zhang, MD
Assistant Professor
Department of Ophthalmology and
    Oculoplastics
University of Washington
Seattle, Washington
United States

Sarah Zhang, BS
Medical Student
University of Arizona College of Medicine
Phoenix, Arizona
United States

Ofira Zloto, MD
Consultant
Ophthalmolgy
Sheba Medical Center
Ramat Gan, Israel

PREFACE

Ophthalmic neoplasms range from benign to malignant and life-threatening tumors. Notably, it has grown significantly in the last 50 years. The field of ocular oncology is a multidisciplinary specialty that requires a coordinated team of ocular oncologists, medical oncologists, pathologists, radiologists, and many more.

Timely diagnosis and treatment are of paramount importance in ocular oncology to avoid vision loss, salvage the eye, and minimize morbidity and mortality. There has been a remarkable increase in the availability of imaging techniques to diagnose and monitor ocular tumors, along with an explosion in prognostic markers and a trend toward precision cancer care.

We designed this book as a case review for readers to use as a quick reference and guide to management of patients in clinical practice. The 66 chapters are devoted to tumors ranging from orbit to eyelid to ocular surface and intraocular tumors. We hope that this book also helps students, residents, and fellows further understand the complex specialty of ocular oncology.

The advancements in the field of ocular oncology have been possible because of the dedicated efforts of numerous specialists. We thank our colleagues for sharing their experience and wisdom in these interesting cases. We also thank our patients for allowing us to use their images to educate and help readers diagnose and manage ocular oncology conditions.

Aparna Ramasubramanian, MD
Carol L. Shields, MD

CONTENTS

SECTION 4   Uveal Pigmented Tumors

SECTION 5   Retinoblastoma

SECTION 6   Nonpigmented Posterior Segment Tumors

CLINICAL CASES in OCULAR ONCOLOGY

Eyelid/Orbital Tumors

CHAPTER 1

Eyelid Squamous Cell Carcinoma

Emmanuel Lee Boniao ▪ Gangadhara Sundar

Chronic Unilateral Blepharoconjunctivitis in a 90-Year-Old

HISTORY OF PRESENT ILLNESS

A 90-year-old female patient with a history of diabetes, hypertension, depression, and a 9-month history of "chronic red eyes" was referred for a new-onset fleshy ulcerative lump of the right lower eyelid (Fig. 1.1). She had initially been treated for several months for blepharitis by a general ophthalmologist. Six months prior to consult, she was seen by the cornea service for a "corneal epithelial defect" with "dendritic ulcer" and managed as herpetic keratitis prior to having everting sutures for a presumed cicatricial entropion from chronic blepharoconjunctivitis and referred to our team for a progressive fleshy ulcerative lump of a 1-month duration. Patient was pseudophakic in both eyes, without previous history of trauma or eyelid surgery. The left eye was unremarkable.

Exam

	OD	OS
External exam	Erythematous eyelid margins with loss of lower eyelashes	Normal
	No regional lymphadenopathy	
Visual acuity	20/40	20/30
Intraocular pressure (mm Hg)	10	14
Sclera/conjunctiva	Diffuse conjunctival injection	White and quiet
Cornea	Diffuse vascularization with central corneal epithelial defect	Clear
Anterior chamber	Mild hazy view	Deep and quiet
Iris	Unremarkable	Unremarkable
	Brown iris, round pupil, no iris neovascularization	Brown iris, pupil round, no iris neovascularization
Lens	Pseudophakic	Pseudophakic
Anterior vitreous	Clear	Clear
Retina/optic nerve	Normal optic nerve, posterior and peripheral retina	Normal optic nerve, posterior and peripheral retina

QUESTIONS TO ASK

- Was there any response to the initial treatment for the condition of the right eye?
- Was there any complaints about the left eye?
- Was there any pain, numbness, or bleeding related to the lower part of the right eyelid?

No financial interest associated with manuscript. No funding supports.

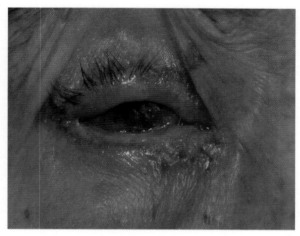

Fig. 1.1 Right eye showing erythema with induration, ulceration, and thickening of eyelid margins with loss of lashes of the lower eyelid. Severe ocular surface disease is also obvious.

- Was there any history of radiation or chronic sun exposure?
- Any long-standing medical history that might be significant, including any organ transplants or immunosuppression?

The patient complained there was no improvement despite multiple treatments for blepharo-conjunctivitis. She did not have any complaints in her left eye. Pain and numbness were absent, but there was a history of bleeding of the right lower eyelid. There was no history of cancer in the family, chronic sun exposure, previous radiation, surgery, chronic medical illness, or medications of concern.

ASSESSMENT

- Inflammatory and infiltrative lesion right lower eyelid with induration, with contiguous extension to the right upper eyelid, cornea, and conjunctiva.

DIFFERENTIAL DIAGNOSIS

- Chronic actinic keratosis
- Chronic diffuse meibomian gland dysfunction with inflammation
- Cutaneous squamous cell carcinoma
- Sebaceous gland carcinoma
- Merkel cell carcinoma
- Basal cell carcinoma—pagetoid type

WORKING DIAGNOSIS

- Cutaneous squamous cell carcinoma of the right lower eyelid

INVESTIGATION AND TESTING

- Incision biopsy of the medial canthal lump and suspicious parts of the lower eyelid

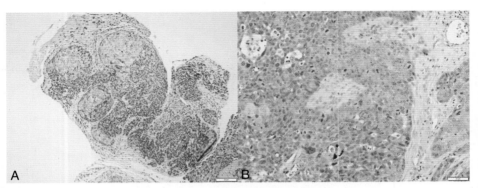

Fig. 1.2 (A) Microscopic image of poorly differentiated squamous cell carcinoma associated with severe squamous dysplasia on the surface epithelium. Hematoxylin and eosin (200x magnification). (B) Poorly differentiated squamous cell carcinoma: geographic islands of malignant squamous cells with severe nuclear pleomorphism, prominent nucleoli, eosinophilic cytoplasm, and brisk mitotic activity. Hematoxylin and eosin (200x magnification).

- All specimens sent for histopathology revealed poorly differentiated squamous cell carcinoma, with severe nuclear pleomorphism, and prominent nucleoli exhibiting brisk mitotic activity (Fig. 1.2).

MANAGEMENT

- Patient and family were offered excision biopsy under frozen section control with primary reconstruction. However, the patient and the family declined any surgical intervention.
- Patient was offered chemotherapy and immunotherapy but declined.
- Patient was offered topical 5% imiquimod cream for skin lesion and 0.04% mitomycin C eye drops for the right eye to which the patient agreed.

FOLLOW-UP

- Patient underwent monthly follow-up with symptomatic treatment with lubricants and intermittent antibiotic-steroid drops. While the erythema transiently improved, there was progressive increase in induration and infiltration over 3 months (Fig. 1.3) with a large mass lesion noted 9 months post-biopsy (Fig. 1.4). The patient was offered surgical intervention at every follow-up and even palliative radiotherapy later, but declined at every stage and eventually succumbed to the disease 1 year later from systemic metastasis.

Key Points

- Malignant epithelial neoplasms of the periocular area in its early stages, especially when presenting with ulceration, may mimic benign conditions such as chronic blepharitis.
- Apart from chronic blepharoconjunctivitis, eyelid and periocular squamous cell carcinoma may be indistinguishable from poorly differentiated sebaceous gland carcinoma by histopathology but may be differentiated by microRNA expression.
- Presentation of eyelid malignancies may be variable and sometimes without pathognomonic features. However, disruption of tissue architecture, loss of lashes, ulceration, and induration should be suspicious.
- Chronic sun exposure, age, and chronic immunosuppression are some risk factors for periocular squamous cell carcinoma.

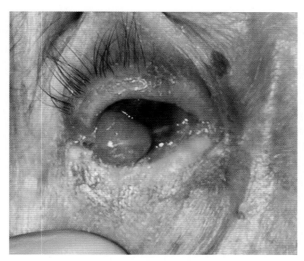

Fig. 1.3 Progressive increase in induration and infiltration of the lesion in the right lower eyelid with nodular growth lateral to the lower eyelid 3 months postbiopsy.

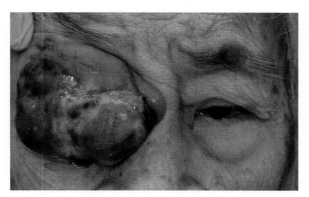

Fig. 1.4 Large ulcerative mass lesion with bleeding involving upper and lower eyelids and obscuration of the globe 9 months after initial presentation.

- Poor prognostic factors for cutaneous squamous cell carcinoma include poor differentiation, chronic immunosuppression, perineural invasion, and orbital invasion.
- Perineural invasion is a form of metastatic spread that may extend to the cavernous sinus and the brain. Its presence is indicative of aggressive behavior and is associated with higher rates of recurrence. Radiotherapy and, more recently, immunotherapy are recommended for these patients.
- Management of locally advanced cutaneous squamous cell carcinoma includes wide excision with frozen section control. Adjunctive cryotherapy, chemotherapy, and/or immunotherapy are also available.
- Immunotherapy with pembrolizumab and cemiplimab may be used for patients with locally advanced disease who are not good candidates for surgery and/or chemotherapy.
- In cases where palliative care is necessary, surgical debulking and/or radiotherapy may be given to lessen disease burden and relieve pain.

- A multidisciplinary team that may consist of oncology, radiation oncology, plastic surgery, and ophthalmology is ideal in managing locally advanced cutaneous squamous cell carcinoma of the periocular region.

Acknowledgment

Pathology contributions from:
Dr. Noel Chia and Dr. Derrick Wen Quan Lian
Department of Pathology
National University Hospital
National University of Singapore
Singapore

CHAPTER 2

Eyelid Basal Cell Carcinoma

Roxana Fu ■ Matthew M. Zhang

Multiple Eyelid Lesions in a 43-Year-Old White Female

HISTORY OF PRESENT ILLNESS

A 43-year-old White female presents for "white" bumps on her right and left lower eyelids. Lesions are painless, without discharge or bleeding, and have been present for about a year.

Exam

	OD	OS
Visual acuity	20/30	20/20
IOP	10 mm Hg	10 mm Hg
Lids/lashes	Right lower eyelid irregular marginal lesion and adjacent madarosis	Left lower lid, white, cystic marginal lesion with posterior conjunctival extension
	Right upper eyelid inclusion cyst	
Sclera/conjunctiva	White and quiet	White and quiet
Cornea	Clear	Clear
AC	Deep and quiet	Deep and quiet
Iris	Normal	Normal
Lens	Trace cortical cataract	Trace cortical cataract
Anterior vitreous	Clear	Clear

AC, Anterior chamber; *IOP*, intraocular pressure.

QUESTIONS TO ASK

- Do you have any personal or family history of cancer?
- Do you have any personal risk factors for developing skin cancer?
- Do you have any other relevant medical history?

The patient has a history of right cheek basal cell carcinoma (BCC) and maxillary odontogenic keratocysts. No history of radiation or immunomodulating therapy. She denies any family history of malignancies.

ASSESSMENT

- Right lower eyelid: irregular posterior eyelid margin lesion with adjacent madarosis (Fig. 2.1)
- Left lower eyelid: tarsal cyst (Fig. 2.2)

No financial interest associated with the manuscript. No funding supports.

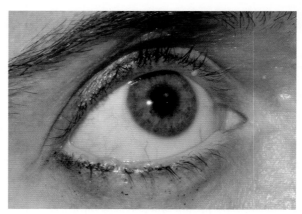

Fig. 2.1 Right eye showing right lower eyelid irregular marginal lesion with madarosis just anterior to the lesion. An incidental right upper eyelid inclusion cyst is seen medially.

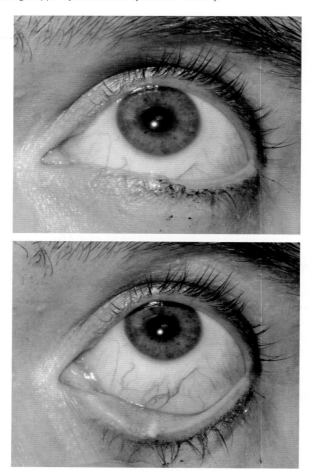

Fig. 2.2 Left eye showing white, cystic, posterior marginal lesion *(top)*. Upon eyelid eversion, posterior palpebral conjunctival extension is demonstrated *(bottom)*.

DIFFERENTIAL DIAGNOSIS

- Right lower eyelid nevus with incidental left lower eyelid tarsal cyst
- Right lower eyelid BCC with incidental left lower eyelid tarsal cyst
- Basal cell nevus syndrome (previously known as Gorlin-Goltz syndrome)

WORKING DIAGNOSIS

- BCC with incidental tarsal cyst, with concern for basal cell nevus syndrome

INVESTIGATION AND TESTING

- Biopsy of suspected BCC and removal of tarsal cyst
- Histopathology revealed basaloid epithelial cells with palisading nuclei consistent with nodular-type BCC of the right lower eyelid
- Cystic lesion with keratinizing stratified squamous epithelium consistent with a tarsal epithelial cyst of the left lower eyelid (Fig. 2.3).

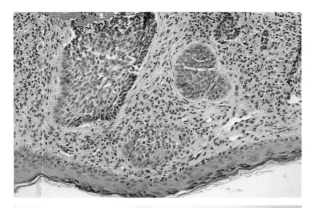
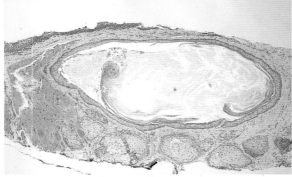

Fig. 2.3 200x light microscopy photograph of the right lower eyelid biopsy specimen showing well-circumscribed lobules of basaloid epithelial cells with palisading nuclei and mitotic figures indicative of nodular-type basal cell carcinoma *(top)*; 20x light microscopy photograph of the left lower eyelid biopsy specimen showing a cystic lesion of tarsus with keratinizing stratified squamous epithelium lacking a granular keratohyaline layer indicative of tarsal epithelial cyst *(bottom)*.

MANAGEMENT

- Patient underwent excision of the right lower eyelid BCC with intraoperative frozen sections.

FOLLOW-UP

- BCC was completely excised with clear margins, and the patient has been established with genetic, dermatology, and ophthalmology clinics for continued surveillance.

Key Points

- BCC, tarsal cyst, and odontogenic keratocyst are known presentations of basal cell nevus syndrome. Among BCC patients, 1 in 200 have basal cell nevus syndrome. It is associated with the Patched1 *(PTCH1)* gene mutation on chromosome 9p22.3, which plays a role in activating the sonic hedgehog (SHH) pathway.
- Additional manifestations include skeletal, central nervous system, cardiac, renal, and gastrointestinal abnormalities. Ophthalmic findings include exophthalmos, rotary nystagmus, strabismus, chalazia, microphthalmia, congenital cataracts, orbital cysts, and colobomas of the choroid, iris, and optic nerve. Therefore, diagnosis and initial screening consist of a full physical examination; genetic, dermatology, and ophthalmology consults with x-rays; MRI brain; cardiac echo; and genetic testing for detection of *PTCH1* mutation.
- Excision of BCC in these patients remains the mainstay of treatment, while radiotherapy is avoided given their predilection for developing neoplasms. Continued management includes close surveillance of the patient and direct family members and UV protection. Vismodegib targets the SHH pathway and can play a role in decreasing and preventing BCCs and odontogenic cysts, and it can be considered for locally advanced, unresectable, or widespread BCC. Patient selection and duration of treatment with vismodegib are ongoing areas of study.
- The prognosis for these patients is generally good with similar life expectancy when there's early defection of BCC and other neoplasms.

CHAPTER 3

Eyelid Melanoma

Bhupendra C.K. Patel ■ John Bladen ■ Raman Malhotra ■ André Litwin

Eyelid Malignant Melanoma in a 47-Year-Old Female of Hispanic Origin

HISTORY OF PRESENT ILLNESS

A previously healthy 47-year-old female presents with a history of having had a pigmented lesion on her right lower eyelid for more than 10 years with little change until 6 months before presentation when she noticed a darkening and enlargement of the lesion.

The patient had seen her primary care physician, who had referred her to a dermatologist who saw her 6 months prior to her presentation to us: she was told it was a pigmented lesion of no concern. There was no photographic documentation of what it looked like at the time, but according to the patient, the lesion was "similar in appearance but had grown since then." She also noticed that the density of the eyelashes had decreased over the previous 6 months.

Exam

	OD	OS
Visual acuity	20/20	20/20
Intra ocular pressure (IOP) (mm Hg)	14	16
Sclera/conjunctiva	White and quiet	White and quiet
Cornea	Clear	Clear
Anterior chamber (AC)	Deep and quiet	Deep and quiet
Lower eyelid anterior	Pigmented lesion 14 mm x 9 mm with dark elevated areas inferiorly (Fig. 3.1)	Normal
Eyelid margin	Pigment affecting the eyelid margin, including the mucocutaneous junction of the right lower eyelid	Normal
Eyelashes	Decreased density of lashes in the region of the pigmented lesion	Normal
Lymph nodes	No palpable lymph nodes	No palpable lymph nodes

QUESTIONS TO ASK

- Where did you grow up?
- Were you exposed to sunlight without protection growing up?
- Have you had any other pigmented lesions on the body in the past?
- Is there a family history of skin cancers?

No financial interest associated with manuscript. Supported in part by an Unrestricted Grant from Research to Prevent Blindness, Inc., New York, NY, to the Department of Ophthalmology & Visual Sciences, University of Utah.

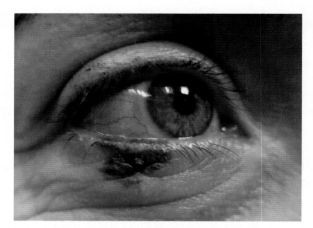

Fig. 3.1 Pigmented lesion right lower eyelid with madarosis, involvement of the lower eyelid skin, the muco-cutaneous junction, and the anterior eyelid margin with no conjunctival involvement.

The patient grew up in Mexico City where she "played out in the sun all the time" and did not use sunscreen or sunglasses until she was an adult and had moved to the United States. She was not aware of any other pigmented lesions on her body, and there was no family history of skin malignancy.

ASSESSMENT

- Pigmented lesion right lower eyelid with madarosis, involvement of the lower eyelid skin, the mucocutaneous junction, and the anterior eyelid margin with no conjunctival involvement
- Raised darker areas inferiorly

DIFFERENTIAL DIAGNOSIS

- Lentigo maligna
- Lentigo maligna melanoma
- Lentigo maligna invasive melanoma

WORKING DIAGNOSIS

- Right lower eyelid lentigo maligna invasive melanoma

INVESTIGATION AND TESTING

- Biopsy confirmed that this was invasive melanoma in the presence of an eyelid lentigo maligna (Fig. 3.2A–B).
- Scintigraphy and lymph node biopsy were negative.

MANAGEMENT

- Patient underwent a Slow Mohs resection of the right lower eyelid melanoma.
- Histopathology confirmed an invasive melanoma in the presence of a lentigo maligna (Fig. 3.3).

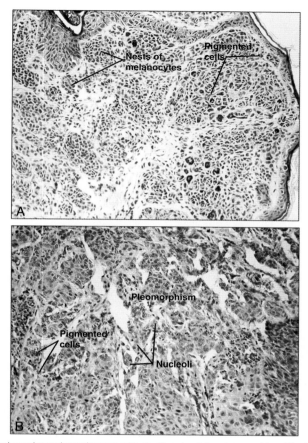

Fig. 3.2 Histopathology showed a melanoma with significant cellular pleomorphism (A) with large nuclei and prominent eosinophilic macronucleoli (B).

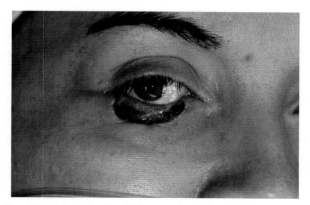

Fig. 3.3 Size of the defect after slow Mohs resection of the right lower eyelid melanoma.

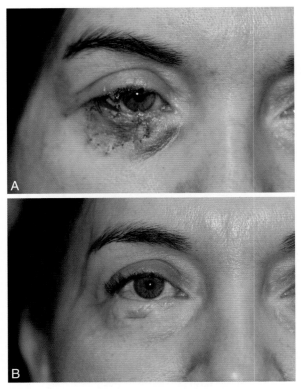

Fig. 3.4 (A) Appearance of the right lower eyelid 5 days after reconstruction of the lower eyelid defect. (B) Appearance of the right lower eyelid 4 years after reconstruction of the lower eyelid defect.

■ Reconstruction with a lateral canthoplasty and full-thickness skin graft was performed (Fig. 3.4A).

FOLLOW-UP

■ The patient was seen every 4 months for 5 years with no recurrence of tumor (Fig. 3.4B).

Key Points

■ Cutaneous melanomas usually arise from melanocytes at the dermal-epidermal junction in normal skin or in a preexisting nevus.
■ One case of eyelid melanoma will be diagnosed for every 50 cases of cutaneous melanomas of the head and neck region. Head and neck melanomas have the highest mortality, with the eyelid representing the worst prognosis with a 10-year mortality of 90%.
■ Eyelid melanomas are divided into melanoma in situ and invasive melanoma.
■ In situ melanomas begin as light brown macules that slowly enlarge over years and may range in size from a few millimeters to over 4 cm. If there is change in size and color, biopsy is indicated. The larger the macule, the higher the chance that an occult melanoma exists.
■ The majority of malignant melanomas of the periorbita involve the lower eyelid (57%). The upper eyelid is involved in 13%, the lateral canthus 10%, and the medial canthus 2%, with the rest involving the brow (13%).

- Risk factors of melanoma include ultraviolet light exposure, previous sunburns, history of nonmelanoma skin cancer, advancing age, family history, and genetic predisposition (including syndromes such as xeroderma pigmentosum).
- The Breslow measure of thickness of the tumor measures thickness from the top of the granular layer of the epidermis to the deepest portion of the melanoma, with measurements recorded to the nearest 0.2 mm thickness.
- The most common histologic subtypes observed in invasive eyelid melanoma are superficial spreading melanoma (35%), lentigo maligna melanoma (31%), and nodular melanoma (19%).
- The ABCDE checklist of pigmented lesions is useful in assessing all pigmented lesions: **A**symmetry, **B**order irregularity, **C**olor changes, **D**iameter more than 6 mm, **E**levation and **E**volution over time.
- Diagnosis requires a full-thickness skin biopsy as the Breslow score is useful in determining prognosis.
- For melanomas in general, the guidelines for resection are 0.5 cm margins for melanoma in situ, 1 cm for lesions <1 mm in depth, 1–2 cm for lesions 1–2 mm thick, and 2–3 cm for thicker lesions. However, these margins are not applicable to eyelid melanomas.
- The eyelid melanoma working group has suggested that margins of 5 mm are adequate for periocular melanomas, although tumors thicker than 1 mm warrant a wider excision. These guidelines are based on consensus and not on any proper studies.
- Margin-controlled excision using the Slow Mohs technique for eyelid melanomas (melanoma antigen is recognized by T1 cells immunostaining) has been recommended with the explanation to the patient that further resection may be necessary to obtain tumor clearance. The Johnson square procedure (where serial peripheral sections are removed for margin control) is another method used to achieve complete clearance of tumor.
- Ninety percent of metastases after treatment of melanoma occur within 5 years.
- Five-year overall survival of eyelid melanoma has been shown to be 77% to 88% for invasive disease and 74% to 89% for melanoma in situ.
- For invasive melanoma survival, poor prognosis is associated with age (more than 75 years) at diagnosis, stage T4, lymph node involvement, and nodular melanoma histologic subtype.
- Local recurrence after treatment of eyelid melanoma has been shown to be 25%, with all the recurrences occurring within the first 5 years. Based on this, 5 years of surveillance is suggested for patients who have undergone eyelid melanoma resection.
- Genetic testing of the tumor involves the identification of *BRAF* or *NRAS*, which can allow access to *BRAF* inhibitors (vemurafenib, dabrafenib, and encorafenib) or *MEK* inhibitors (trametinib, binimetinib, selumetinib, cobimetinib). Approximately 50% of all cutaneous melanomas harbor *BRAF* mutations.
- Checkpoint inhibitor immunotherapy is independent of the tumor's genetic profile. Drugs such as nivolumab may be used for patients with recurrence.
- Sentinel lymph node biopsy is recommended for patients with T2a disease or T1b disease with lymphovascular invasion and/or mitotic rate of more than 2 mm^2.
- Vitamin D levels need to be monitored, as it has been shown that high-circulating vitamin D concentration is associated with reduced melanoma progression and improved survival.

CHAPTER 4

Orbit Infantile Hemangioma

Elizabeth Dupuy

Increased Swelling of the Eyelid in a 2-Month-Old Child

HISTORY OF PRESENT ILLNESS

A previously healthy 2-month-old male presented with a complaint of eyelid swelling. His mother noted the eyelid swelling at 7 days of life and reports that it has progressively worsened. There was no trauma. There was no pain or tearing.

Exam

On visual inspection, there was mild lid ptosis (Fig. 4.1A) and swelling of the left eyelid with a subtle blue discoloration (Fig. 4.1B). The eyelid was slightly warm and soft on palpation.

Exam

On visual inspection, there was mild lid ptosis (Fig. 4.1A) and swelling of the left eyelid with a subtle blue discoloration (Fig. 4.1B). The eyelid was slightly warm and soft on palpation.

	OD	OS
Visual acuity	Fix and follow vision (F&F)	F&F
IOP	Finger tension normal	Finger tension normal
Eyelid	Normal	Ptosis left upper eyelid 0.5 mm with hemangioma
Sclera/conjunctiva	White	White
Cornea	Clear	Clear
AC	Quiet	Quiet
Iris	Normal	Normal
Lens	Clear	Clear
Anterior vitreous	Clear	Clear
Retina/optic nerve	Normal	Normal

AC, Anterior chamber; IOP, intraocular pressure.

QUESTIONS TO ASK

- Does the child have any birthmarks or other skin lesions?
- Were there complications to the pregnancy?
- Does the child have any other relevant past medical history?

The patient does have one small pink birthmark on the arm. The pregnancy was complicated by gestational hypertension. The patient was born prematurely at 34 weeks. Parents deny any other significant past medical history.

No financial interest associated with the manuscript. No funding supports.

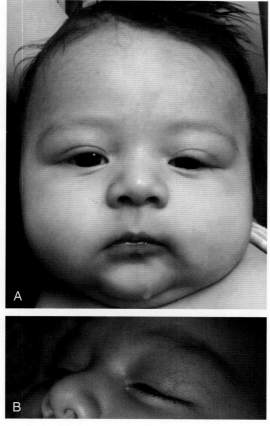

Fig. 4.1 (A) On close inspection, a slight blue hue is visible. (B) A deep hemangioma of the eyelid presenting with swelling and ptosis.

ASSESSMENT

- Soft tissue mass, OS

DIFFERENTIAL DIAGNOSIS

- Orbit infantile hemangioma (orbit capillary hemangioma)
- Congenital hemangioma
- Rhabdomyosarcoma
- Metastatic neuroblastoma
- Lymphatic or venous malformation
- Chalazion, hordeolum

WORKING DIAGNOSIS

- Orbit infantile hemangioma (orbit capillary hemangioma), OS

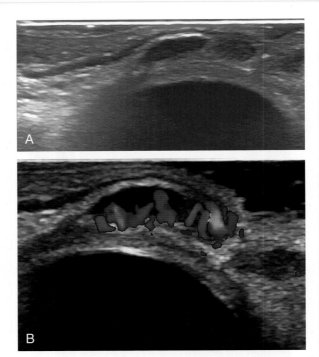

Fig. 4.2 (A) Ultrasound demonstrates two well-defined hypoechoic nodules in the subcutaneous tissue. (B) On color Doppler, ultrasound shows high vascular density.

INVESTIGATION AND TESTING

- Soft tissue ultrasound showed two contiguous ovoid hypoechoic structures in the upper eyelid measuring 6.2 × 5.3 × 2.2 mm and 5.2 × 3.9 × 2.8 mm (Fig. 4.2A). Both lesions demonstrate significant vascularity. Doppler assessment demonstrates both arterial and venous flow within the lesions, most likely representing hemangiomas (Fig. 4.2B).

MANAGEMENT

- The patient was referred to treatment with an oral beta blocker: propranolol.

FOLLOW-UP

- There was improvement in the size and color within 1 week of treatment initiation.
- The patient did well with periodic follow-up to titrate the dose of medication based on weight gain.
- The patient was monitored for the development of visual axis obstruction and amblyopia.

KEY POINTS

- Recognized by the International Society for the Study of Vascular Anomalies (ISSVA) as infantile hemangioma, although the term *orbit capillary hemangioma* predominates in ophthalmology literature.
- Other names include infantile periocular hemangioma, juvenile hemangioma, hemangioblastoma, and strawberry nevus of infancy.

- Very common benign vascular tumors can appear anywhere on the skin and subcutaneous tissue, including the eyelid and orbit.
- Benign vascular tumors are more common among patients with certain risk factors, including female sex, non-Hispanic White race, prematurity, low birth weight, and twins. Prenatal associations include preeclampsia, placental abnormalities, and advanced maternal age.
- Physical exam:
  - Superficial hemangiomas are pink vascular papules or plaques (Fig. 4.3A–B).

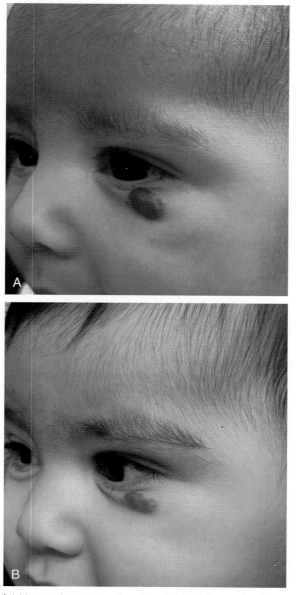

Fig. 4.3 (A) A superficial hemangioma presenting with a bright pink vascular plaque on the lower eyelid. (B) The same lesion 6 months after treatment with oral propranolol.

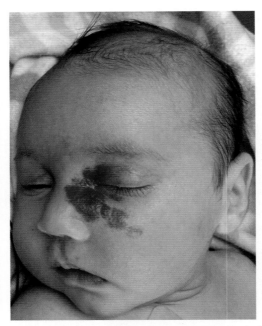

Fig. 4.4 A superficial lesion in a segmental pattern in a patient under evaluation for PHACES syndrome.

- ■ Deep hemangiomas are skin-colored or bluish subcutaneous nodules. Hemangioma deep in the orbit can present with proptosis without skin findings.
- ■ Mixed or combined hemangiomas have both superficial and deep features.
- ■ Involvement of the conjunctiva or the presence of other hemangiomas on the skin may be diagnostic clues.
- ■ Infantile hemangiomas are usually not fully formed at birth and become apparent in the first weeks of life.
- ■ Infantile hemangiomas have a characteristic growth pattern comprised of a rapid growth phase, slow growth phase, and involution phase.
  - ■ The rapid growth phase is usually complete in the first few months of life, and growth is altogether completed by 12 to 18 months of life.
  - ■ The involution phase occurs slowly over several years.
- ■ Biopsy is rarely required to establish a diagnosis. Tissue will stain positively for glucose transporter 1 (GLUT-1), whereas congenital hemangiomas (lesions that are fully developed at birth) will be GLUT-1 negative.
- ■ Posterior fossa anomaly, hemangioma, arterial anomaly, cardiac defect, eye anomaly, sternal cleft or supraumbilical raphe (PHACES) syndrome can be found in infants with large segmental hemangiomas of the face. Patients should be referred for further evaluation if this is suspected (Fig. 4.4).
- ■ Treatment is not warranted for all hemangiomas; it should be considered in cases leading to cosmetic disfigurement, amblyopia due to visual axis obstruction or anisometropia, significant proptosis, or when skin ulceration occurs.
- ■ Oral and topical beta blockers are the treatment of choice.
- ■ Other treatments include intralesional or systemic steroids; treatments such as radiation, interferon, and others have fallen out of favor.
- ■ Surgery is reserved for large vision-threatening lesions.

IMAGING

- Ultrasound:
  - Echogenic well-defined mass
  - Color Doppler ultrasound will show vascular flow into the lesion.
- Magnetic resonance imaging (MRI):
  - The lesions are hypointense relative to orbital fat and isointense to muscle on T1- and iso- to hyperintense on T2-weighted images. The lesions demonstrate diffuse enhancement, which is to be best appreciated with fat-suppressed images. Flow voids may be present within the lesion.

CHAPTER 5

Orbital Dermoid Cyst

Azzam Malkawi ■ S. Elizabeth Dugan ■ Nicole West ■ Christopher Compton

Painless, Slow-Growing, Periorbital Mass in a 3-Year-Old Child

HISTORY OF PRESENT ILLNESS

A 3-year-old female presents with left eyelid swelling. Her parents report it has been present since birth, and they express concern for its appearance. She has no prior ocular or medical history and no trauma to either eye.

Exam

	OD	OS
Visual acuity	20/20	20/20
IOP (mm Hg)	15	15
Eyelids/lashes	Normal	Painless, smooth, flesh-colored mass palpable in superficial temporal orbital region, mobile under skin but fixed to periosteum (Fig. 5.1)
Sclera/conjunctiva	White and quiet	White and quiet
Cornea	Clear	Clear
AC	Deep and quiet	Deep and quiet
Iris	Unremarkable	Unremarkable
	Brown iris, pupil round	Brown iris, pupil round
Lens	Clear	Clear
Anterior vitreous	Clear	Clear
Retina/optic nerve	Normal optic nerve, posterior and peripheral retina	Normal optic nerve, posterior and peripheral retina

AC, Anterior chamber; *IOP,* intraocular pressure.

QUESTIONS TO ASK

- When did you first notice this mass, and how has it changed over time?
- Any bulging eyes, drooping eyelids, double vision, or pain or difficulty with looking in different directions?
- Any bulging of eyes with chewing food?

The patient's parents first noticed this mass at birth. It started as a 1-cm mass and has slowly grown to 3 cm in diameter. The patient's parents have never noticed any proptosis, ptosis, extraocular movement restriction, diplopia, or proptosis with mastication.

No financial interest is associated with the manuscript. No funding support.

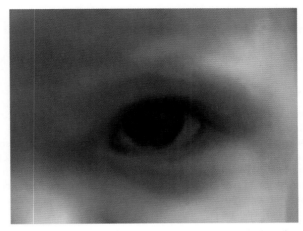

Fig. 5.1 External photograph showing the dermoid cyst near the lateral eyebrow.

ASSESSMENT

Painless well-defined mass that is compressible, smooth, and mobile in the superficial temporal orbital region, near the lateral eyebrow.

DIFFERENTIAL DIAGNOSIS

- Epidermoid cyst (epidermal inclusion)
- Trichilemmal cyst
- Pilomatrixoma
- Lymphatic malformation
- Lipoma
- Teratoma
- Congenital cystic eye
- Colobomatous cyst
- Lacrimal gland tumor
- Congenital encephalocele
- Dacryocele
- Mucocele

WORKING DIAGNOSIS

- Superficial dermoid cyst in temporal periorbital area OS.

INVESTIGATION AND TESTING

- No further imaging or testing is needed for superficial dermoid cysts.
- Deep dermoid cysts need imaging to evaluate their extent into bony structures before surgical excision. This step can help with surgical planning.
- Computed tomography (CT) will show a round or ovoid soft tissue mass with an enhancing wall and a nonenhancing lumen.

- Magnetic resonance imaging (MRI) will show a well-defined round or ovoid lesion with variable signal intensity in the lumen, depending on the homogeneity or heterogeneity of the mass.
- Ultrasound will show a well-defined homogenous and hypoechoic cystic lesion.

MANAGEMENT

- Complete surgical excision without rupture is indicated because these cysts tend to leak their irritating contents into surrounding tissues.
- All traces of epithelium must be excised. If accidentally ruptured, it is necessary to irrigate copiously with saline and ensure that the capsule has been removed entirely. If any epithelium remains, it secretes an irritant that induces orbital inflammation and allows for cyst recurrence.
- These recurrent dermoid cysts can lead to infection, abscess formation, and fibrosis. Additionally, remaining inflammation can cause an orbitocutaneous fistula or a granulomatous-type inflammatory reaction in the case of rupture.

FOLLOW-UP

- The incision healed well without any complications.
- The pathology was consistent with dermoid cyst (Figs. 5.2 and 5.3).
- The patient did not require any further treatment and remained stable during follow-up.

KEY POINTS

- Dermoid cysts are a type of congenital choristoma that consists of keratinized epithelium, hair follicles, and glandular tissue. They are benign cutaneous growths that occur due to entrapment of epithelial tissue during development, and they are the most common orbital tumor in childhood.

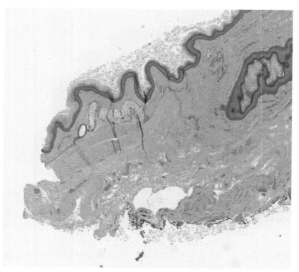

Fig. 5.2 Low-power view of dermoid cyst wall structure in cross-section. The cyst is lined by normal stratified squamous epithelium. The *blue* ink on the periphery delineates the surgical margin. The middle of the cyst is filled with keratin and hair shafts.

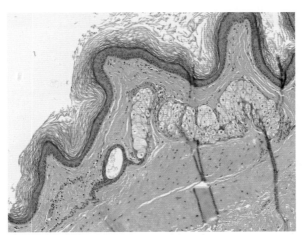

Fig. 5.3 Adnexal structures of dermoid cyst. The cyst wall has adnexal structures present, and this feature differentiates them from epidermal inclusion cysts. For example, the sebaceous glands are associated with the hair follicle cut in cross-section on the left.

- The superotemporal angle is the most common site in the orbit because these cysts are located along lines of embryonic fusion, such as the frontozygomatic suture and the lower end of the coronal suture.
- Superficial dermoid cysts present as painless well-defined cystic masses that are compressible, smooth, and mobile.
- The symptomatology of deep dermoid cysts is dependent on mass effect and their location in the orbit. They generally present in adulthood with a gradually increasing protruding eye or an acutely inflamed orbit due to rupture.
- If proptosis with mastication is present, suspect a dumbbell dermoid cyst. Part of the lesion will be in the orbit, and the other part will be located in the temporal fossa with the bony defect at the suture line connecting the ends.
- Computerized tomography (CT) and MRI can be helpful in elucidating the extent of a dermoid cyst, particularly with bone involvement.
- Both superficial and deep dermoid cysts are treated with en bloc excision. It is important not to rupture the cyst and to excise all epithelium. If any epithelium remains, it secretes an irritant that induces orbital inflammation and allows for cyst recurrence.

CHAPTER 6

Orbit Lymphoma

Sara E. Lally ■ Carol L. Shields

Tearing and Eye Swelling OS for 4 Months in a 54-Year-Old Male

HISTORY OF PRESENT ILLNESS

A 54-year-old male noted eye swelling and tearing left eye for 4 months. Patient thought it was secondary to sinus disease and was seen by his primary doctor. He has no prior ocular history or trauma to either eye.

Exam

	OD	OS
Visual acuity	20/25	20/30
IOP (mm Hg)	12	27
Sclera/conjunctiva	White and quiet, no salmon patch	Dilated vessel temporally, with injection, faint salmon patch, and chemosis
Cornea	Clear	Clear
AC	Deep and quiet	Deep and quiet
Iris	Normal	Normal
	Blue iris, pupil round	Blue iris, pupil round
Lens	Clear	Clear
Anterior vitreous	Clear	Clear
Retina/optic nerve	Normal optic nerve, small juxtapapillary nevus measuring 1.5 × 1.5 × flat with no risk factors	Normal optic nerve with no edema, pallor, or tortuous vessels
		No choroidal folds or loss of choroidal vasculature
External	No enophthalmos, no palpable masses	Fullness of the lower lid, 3 mm of proptosis (no change with Valsalva maneuver), + resistance to retropulsion
Motility	Full	Full
Red desaturation	None	None
Lymph nodes	No preauricular, anterior cervical, submandibular lymphadenopathy	No preauricular, anterior cervical, submandibular lymphadenopathy

AC, Anterior chamber; *IOP,* intraocular pressure.

No financial interest associated with the manuscript. No funding supports.

QUESTIONS TO ASK

- Any pain or double vision? Notice any redness of the eyes?
- Any systemic medications, especially any immune-modulating medications?
- Any past medical history of autoimmune conditions, cancer, or trauma?

The patient has never complained of pain or double vision. No signs of redness in both eyes. He is not on any systemic medication. The patient denies any significant past medical history.

ASSESSMENT

- Fullness of the lower lid with a palpable mass inferotemporally and 3 mm of proptosis on the left, OS; motility was full (Fig. 6.1).

DIFFERENTIAL DIAGNOSIS

- Thyroid orbitopathy
- Lymphoma
- Idiopathic orbital inflammation
- Metastasis

WORKING DIAGNOSIS

- Orbital lymphoma OS

INVESTIGATION AND TESTING

- MRI revealed diffuse enlargement of the left lateral rectus muscle and molding of the lesion to the globe (Fig. 6.2).
- Ultrasound showed no thickening of the choroid or extraocular extension. Ultrasound biomicroscopy (UBM) showed no ciliary body enlargement.

MANAGEMENT

- Patient underwent orbitotomy on the left side. The left lateral rectus muscle was not involved.
- Histopathology revealed orbital tissue with diffuse infiltration of well-differentiated lymphoid cells. Germinal centers were not evident. Cells were CD20 positive. Findings were consistent with MALT lymphoma (Fig. 6.3).

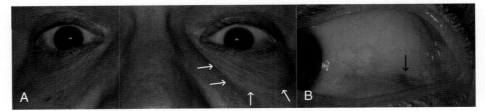

Fig. 6.1   (A) External photograph revealing fullness of the lower lid *(white arrows)* and 3 mm of proptosis on the left, OS. (B) Chemosis, faint salmon patch, and dilated tortuous vessel is noted *(black arrow)*.

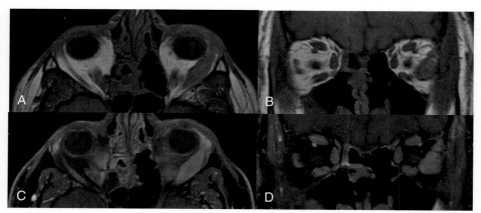

Fig. 6.2 (A and C) MRI revealed diffuse enlargement of the lateral rectus muscle and molding of the lesion to the globe on axial cut. On T1-weighted sequences, the muscle is similar in signal intensity compared to the remaining extraocular muscles. (B) On coronal cut, the enlargement appears to involve the inferior aspect of the muscle belly. (D) With fat suppression, lesion appears separate from the lateral rectus muscle.

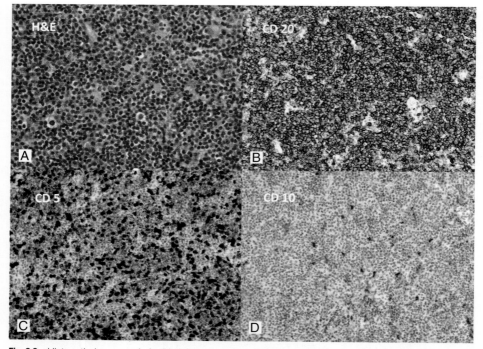

Fig. 6.3 Histopathology revealed orbital tissue largely replaced by sheets of (A) small and well-differentiated lymphoid cells that were (B) CD20 positive, (C) CD5 negative, and (D) CD10 negative, and thereby compatible with MALT lymphoma.

FOLLOW-UP

- The patient underwent a full systemic workup, which was negative. He underwent stereotactic radiotherapy to the left orbit.
- MRI scans and systemic monitoring were recommended.
- Three years after initial diagnosis, the patient was diagnosed with lymphoma of the left maxilla. Radiotherapy was performed.

KEY POINTS

- Orbital lymphoma is the most common primary tumor in older adults.
- The most common type of orbital lymphoma is extranodal marginal zone lymphoma (MALT), followed by follicular lymphoma (FL), diffuse large B-cell lymphoma (DLBCL), and mantle cell lymphoma (MCL). MALT and FL have good life prognosis, whereas DLBCL and MCL have worse life prognosis. Natural killer/T-cell (NK/T) lymphomas are extremely rare.
- The etiology is unknown; however, it is felt to be multifactorial. Infectious, inflammatory, and autoimmune factors have been proposed.
- In patients with orbital lymphoma alone, one-third will develop systemic disease at 10 years. Those with bilateral orbital disease have a higher chance (75% at 10 years) of developing systemic involvement.
- Radiation is the gold standard for treatment. However, options include observation, antibiotics, surgery, radiation, systemic therapy, or intralesional injections.

CHAPTER 7

Orbit Cavernous Venous Malformation

Usha Singh ▪ Khushdeep Abhaypal ▪ Manu Saini

Right Lower Eyelid Swelling, Inferior Orbital Mass, Proptosis and Globe Displacement in a 58-Year-Old Female

HISTORY OF PRESENT ILLNESS

A previously healthy 58-year-old female presented with right lower eyelid swelling. She was asymptomatic 10 years ago when she noticed swelling that was gradually increasing in size. It was painless, as well as progressive without causing any functional deficit.

She complained that her eye had a forward bulge and that her eyeball was pushed up, more so during the last 8 months (Fig. 7.1). It had started hampering her side vision. However, there was no decrease in vision or diplopia. There was no prior ocular history or trauma to the eye.

Exam

	OD	OS
Visual acuity	6/9	6/6
IOP (mm Hg)	19	17
Pupils	No RAPD	No RAPD
Proptosis (exophthalmometry)	26 mm	22 mm
Globe displacement	Forward and superonasal	Normal
Extraocular motility	Mild restriction of motility in lateral and inferior gaze	No restriction
Color	No redness of overlying skin	Within normal limits
Eyelid	Lid laxity of upper and lower eyelid	Lid laxity of upper and lower eyelid
	Upper lid: dermatochalasis, superior sulcus fullness present	Upper lid: dermatochalasis
	Lower lid: fat bulge medially, swelling over lateral lower lid, overlying skin freely mobile	Lower lid: within normal limits
Mass site	Inferior orbit	Nil
Palpation		
Touch	Firm to soft, partially compressible	Nil
Temperature	Normal temperature	Normal temperature
Shape	Round to oval	Within normal limits

No financial interest is associated with the manuscript. No funding support.

Exam—cont'd

	OD	OS
Mass size	Approximately 2 cm × 2 cm anterior surface, posterior extent not palpable	No mass palpable
Fixation to surrounding structures	Nil	Nil
Ballotable	Minimally	Nil
Retrobulbar resistance	Increased	Normal
On retropulsion	On retropulsion of globe, prominence of mass is seen	Normal
Cornea/sclera/conjunctiva	Within normal limits	Within normal limits
Anterior segment	Normal, no Lisch nodules	Normal
Posterior segment	Media clear	Media clear
	Retina and optic disc within normal limits	Retina and optic disc within normal limits
Pulsation	Nil	Nil
Valsalva	Negative	Negative
Schirmer test	15 mm	7 mm
Regional lymph nodes	No lymph nodes palpable	No lymph nodes palpable

IOP, Intraocular pressure; *RAPD,* relative afferent pupil defect.

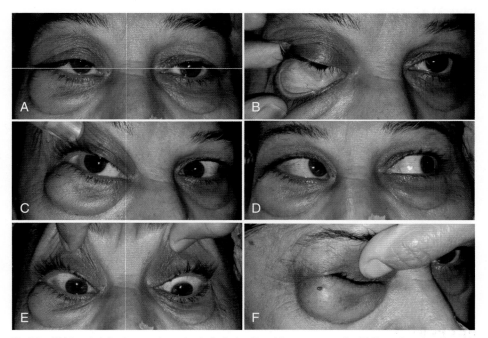

Fig. 7.1 (A) Mass in inferotemporal quadrant displacing the globe superonasally. (B) Normal conjunctiva with no adhesions or congestion. (C) Restricted lateral gaze. (D) Normal medial gaze. (E) Restricted down gaze. (F) On retropulsion, prominence of mass is visible.

QUESTIONS TO ASK

- Do you have any history of injury to your eye?
- Are there any similar masses in your body?
- Does lesion increase in size on bending?

There is no history of trauma to the eye. There are no other similar masses in the body and the mass does not increase on bending.

ASSESSMENT

- Firm to soft palpable mass in the inferotemporal quadrant.

DIFFERENTIAL DIAGNOSIS

- Cavernous venous malformation
- Schwannoma
- Fibrous histiocytoma
- Isolated neurofibroma
- Solitary fibrous tumor

WORKING DIAGNOSIS

- Localized, vascular malformation of the right orbit.

INVESTIGATION AND TESTING

- Contrast-enhanced imaging of the orbit and brain (Fig. 7.2).
- Well-circumscribed heterogenous mass lesion seen in right orbit, primarily occupying extraconal space and abutting and pushing the globe superonasally. It is also pushing the lateral rectus upward. There is no compression on the optic nerve. There is honeycomb appearance of a mass lesion on contrast-enhanced CT scan of orbit. Enhancement pattern is patchy. On contrast-enhanced MRI, a clear distinction is seen between the lateral rectus and the mass lesion.

MANAGEMENT

- Patient underwent anterior orbitotomy via inferolateral skin-crease incision. Sharp and blunt dissection was used with cryoextraction of a red, spongy, vascularized mass lesion. There were no intraoperative complications.
- Histopathology reported circumscribed lesion composed of varied-size blood vessels on low magnification. Higher magnification showed blood vessels of venous caliber lined by flattened endothelium (Fig. 7.3).

FOLLOW-UP

- During a follow-up at 5 months, patient has minimal diplopia in extreme right lateral gaze, likely due to lateral rectus contracture.

KEY POINTS

- Cavernous venous malformation (ISSVA, 2018)—previously called cavernous hemangioma of the orbit—is a common, benign, noninfiltrative, slowly progressive, well-circumscribed, vascular mass presenting in adults.

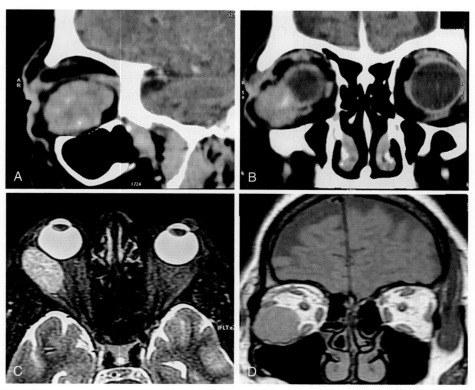

Fig. 7.2 Imaging of the orbits. (A) CT scan shows a heterogenous oval mass lesion in the inferior orbit. (B) Globe indentation by the mass lesion. Both A and B show patchy enhancement. (C) MRI orbit scan shows honeycomb morphology of the well-circumscribed mass lesion. (D) Mass pushing lateral rectus up and away from the optic nerve.

- Most of the time, it is located in the retrobulbar space, thereby presenting as proptosis. Rarely, it can be extraconal, painful, and multiple.
- A common differential diagnosis is schwannoma. Dynamic MRA distinguishes it from schwannoma by the findings of progressive enhancement.
- Surgical resection of the mass is indicated if it causes functional loss. In this case, the mass lesion was big, which was what caused hampering of the lateral visual field.

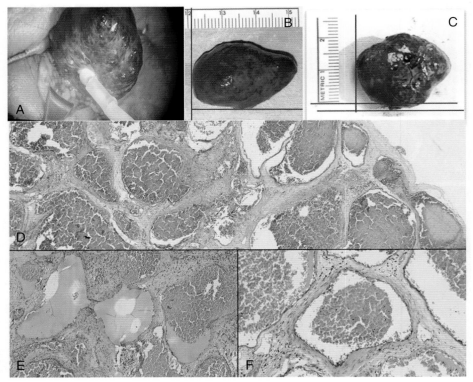

Fig. 7.3 (A) Cryoextraction of vascular mass. (B) Gross specimen measures 3.2 × 2.2 mm. (C) Irregular rough surface that was in contact with globe. (D) Microscopic low magnification showing circumscribed lesion composed of varied-size blood vessels (H&E × 100). (E) Vessels of venous caliber lined by flattened endothelium (H&E × 200). (F) High magnification showing the blood vessels of venous caliber (H&E × 400).

Suggested Reading

ISSVA. Classification; 2018. https://www.issva.org/classification (Accessed 25 August 2023).

CHAPTER 8

Orbit Lymphangioma

Lakshmi Mahesh ■ Smitha Menon

Painful Proptosis in a 5-Year-Old Child

HISTORY OF PRESENT ILLNESS

A 5-year-old female presents with sudden-onset right eye proptosis of 5 days' duration with accompanying pain. She has no prior history of ocular trauma. She gives history of preceding upper respiratory tract infection.

Exam

The child was in pain and was not cooperative for detailed examination of the right eye. Nonaxial proptosis of the right eye was noted. The orbit was tense and tender on palpation, making it difficult to examine the eye (Fig. 8.1A).

Exam

	OD	OS
Visual acuity	Perception of light	6/6
IOP (mm Hg)	Unable to assess	Unable to assess
Lids	Edema, dilated subcutaneous blood vessels seen	Normal
Sclera/conjunctiva	Generalized congestion and inferior chemosis	White and quiet
Cornea	Clear	Clear
AC	Deep and quiet	Deep and quiet
Iris	Brown iris	Brown iris
Pupillary	Round, RAPD 1+	Round, normal reaction to light
Lens	Clear	Clear
Anterior vitreous	Unable to assess	Clear
Retina/optic nerve	Unable to assess	Normal optic nerve, posterior and peripheral retina

AC, Anterior chamber; *IOP,* intraocular pressure; *RAPD,* relative afferent pupil defect.

QUESTIONS TO ASK

- Has your daughter ever had redness or pain in her right eye?
- Has there been any incidence of swelling of the right eye in the past following acute symptoms of sinusitis?
- Any history of recent injury?

No financial interest associated with the manuscript. No funding supports.

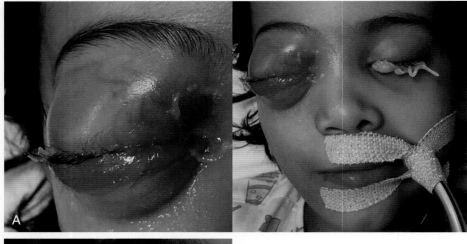

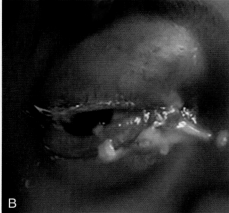

Fig. 8.1 (A) External photograph shows tense orbit with nonaxial proptosis and inferior conjunctival chemosis of the right eye. (B) After two doses of intravenous steroid injection, there was some decrease in the pain and periorbital inflammation, thus making it possible to gently retract the upper eyelid for better examination of the eye.

The patient has never complained of pain in her right eye. There has not been any sign of redness or swelling of the eye in the past. However, she did have symptoms of upper respiratory infection preceding the onset of acute proptosis.

ASSESSMENT

- Painful proptosis, right eye

DIFFERENTIAL DIAGNOSIS

- Lymphangioma
- Cavernous hemangioma
- Orbital hemorrhage
- Arteriovenous fistula

WORKING DIAGNOSIS

- Intraorbital bleed in a case of orbital lymphangioma, right eye

INVESTIGATION AND TESTING

- CT and MRI of the orbits with contrast were done. CT showed an irregular, lobulated lesion with cystic and soft tissue attenuation occupying the intraconal and extraconal regions of the right orbit, resulting in proptosis. A predominantly cystic part of the lesion measuring 3.5 cm × 3.8 cm × 2.7 cm was located superomedial to the eyeball, thus pushing the globe inferolaterally. There was no postcontrast enhancement. No calcification was noted within the lesion. The lesion appeared to be encasing the optic nerve all around. Bony orbital walls appeared normal. MR axial imaging showed a multilobulated intraconal and extraconal lesion surrounding the optic nerve with low to intermediate signals on T1 and high signal on T2 with multiple cystic spaces and fluid-hemorrhage levels.

MANAGEMENT

- The patient was admitted in the hospital and started on intravenous steroids to reduce the periorbital inflammation and mass effect on the optic nerve (Fig. 8.1B).
- She underwent right superomedial orbitotomy with modified Lynch incision under general anesthesia. Multiple chocolate cysts were identified in the superomedial orbit (Fig. 8.2A). Thick altered blood was aspirated. Cyst walls were gently dissected and excised. Good decompression was noted on the table (Fig. 8.2B). The pupil was monitored throughout the surgery. Adequate hemostasis was ensured.
- Histopathology revealed a vasoformative lesion composed of endothelium-lined vascular channels of various luminal diameters filled with blood (venous component) and convoluted collagenous wall-like structures with flattened endothelial cells (lymphatic component). Focal foamy and hemosiderin-laden macrophages were noted.
- The patient was given a short course of oral steroids after the procedure.
- In view of the coexisting vascular component within the lesion, oral propranolol was started after about 1 month postoperatively in consultation with a pediatric cardiologist. Further improvement was noted in the degree of proptosis.

FOLLOW-UP

- The patient has been on regular follow-up for close to a year.
- Unaided vision in the right eye is maintained at 6/9. There is mild residual proptosis. The pupil shows relative afferent pupillary defect (RAPD) 1+ (Fig. 8.3).
- Postoperative MR imaging shows residual lesion that is more in the intraconal compartment with resultant mild proptosis (Figs. 8.4A–B).
- While dealing with the residual tumor in the future, there may be a role for imaging-guided intralesional injection of sclerosants like bleomycin.

KEY POINTS

- Orbital lymphangiomas are multicystic malformations that involve the lymphatic and vascular systems. They occur most commonly in the head and face regions in the pediatric age group. They constitute about 25% of benign pediatric vascular tumors.
- They may be superficial, deep, or combined (with both superficial and deep components) in nature.

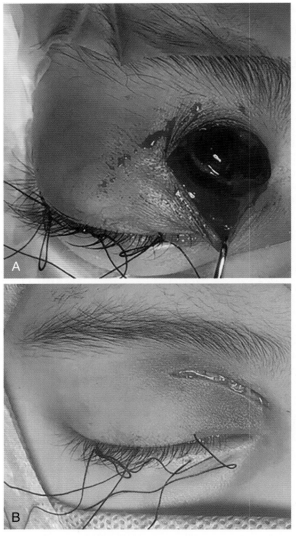

Fig. 8.2 (A) Intraoperative photograph showing right superomedial orbitotomy using a modified Lynch incision with chocolate cyst exposed in the superomedial orbit. (B) Good intraoperative orbital decompression is noted.

- There may be other coexisting vascular malformations in the eye (iris or retina), cheek, palate, or intracranial region.
- Spontaneous intraorbital hemorrhage can cause acute painful proptosis that can be sight-threatening due to resultant corneal exposure or compressive optic neuropathy.
- Observation is recommended in patients with non–vision-threatening lesions.

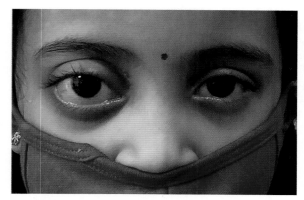

Fig. 8.3 External photograph shows good postoperative decrease in proptosis of the right eye.

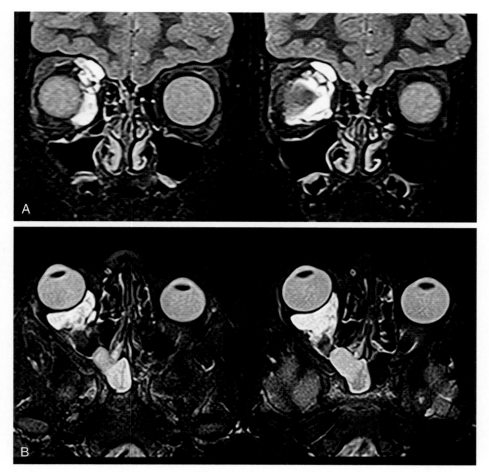

Fig. 8.4 Postoperative (A) MR coronal and (B) axial imaging shows residual lesion in the right orbit that is more in the intraconal compartment with resultant mild proptosis.

- Sclerotherapy with intralesional injection of sclerosants is recommended for macrocystic lesions or after aspiration of chocolate cysts.
- Surgery is challenging owing to the fact that the lesion may be in close proximity to other orbital structures. Hence it is reserved for vision-threatening lesions.
- Regular follow-up for clinical monitoring is necessary. Imaging may be repeated as required.
- Multidisciplinary approach is followed in management of such patients.
- Counseling of the patient and relatives regarding the impact of the lesion on vision, residual lesion, and possible increase of the lesion should be discussed.

CHAPTER 9

Orbit Rhabdomyosarcoma

Hila Goldberg Kremer ■ Bita Esmaeli

Orbital Rhabdomyosarcoma: Assessment of Treatment Response

HISTORY OF PRESENT ILLNESS

An 8-year-old male with a 6-month history of an orbital mass, which had been biopsied and treated as embryonal rhabdomyosarcoma, is currently presenting with residual left eye upper lid swelling and mild proptosis.

Exam

	OD	OS
Visual acuity	20/20	20/20
Pupils (dark, light, react, APD)	4, 3, brisk, none	4, 3, brisk, none
IOP (mm Hg)	Soft (palpation)	Soft (palpation)
External	Normal	Mild proptosis and periorbital edema
Eyelids	Normal	Upper lid swelling
Sclera/conjunctiva	White and quiet	White and quiet
Cornea	Clear	Clear
AC	Deep and quiet	Deep and quiet
Iris	Round and reactive	Round and reactive
Lens	Clear	Clear
Vitreous	Clear	Clear
Disc	Normal 0.3	Normal 0.3
Retina/macula	Normal	Normal

AC, Anterior chamber; *APD,* afferent pupillary defect; *IOP,* intraocular pressure.

QUESTIONS TO ASK

- Does the child have any signs of infection/inflammation such as fever/pain/redness?
- Has the child complained of blurry vision?
- Does the child have any new systemic symptoms or complaints?
- What was the exact chemotherapy regimen and duration? Was radiation therapy given? Did the imaging studies after administration of chemotherapy show the resolution of mass in the orbit?

No financial interest is associated with the manuscript. No funding support.

The patient denies pain in the left eye or elsewhere and does not have blurry vision. There are no systemic complaints, no fever, and no redness/warmth around the eyes.

DIFFERENTIAL DIAGNOSIS

- Recurrent or residual orbital rhabdomyosarcoma
- Dermoid cyst
- Venolymphatic malformation
- Lacrimal gland lesion/tumor
- Optic nerve glioma
- Orbital metastasis

WORKING DIAGNOSIS

- Residual left orbital rhabdomyosarcoma.

INVESTIGATION AND TESTING

- Initial workup (completed in previous facility before starting chemotherapy):
  - Orbital MRI: left orbit superolateral solid mass, measuring 3.4 cm × 2.0 cm × 2.8 cm, T2 hyperintense and strongly enhancing (Fig. 9.1).
  - Bone marrow biopsy: negative.
  - Lumbar puncture (LP): Cerebrospinal fluid (CSF) negative for malignant cells.
  - PET/CT: increased F-fluorodeoxyglucose (FDG) uptake in left orbital mass, no hypermetabolic lymphadenopathy or metastatic disease.
- Pathology review of previous orbital biopsy: embryonal rhabdomyosarcoma with Ki-67 index of 50%; treatment effect/necrosis present in 30%.

MANAGEMENT

- Initial treatment (completed in previous facility after diagnostic biopsy):
  - Chemotherapy with VAC (vincristine/actinomycin/cyclophosphamide) 24-week protocol.
  - Proton radiation therapy (total of 50.4 Gy) given concurrently with chemotherapy
- Halfway treatment evaluation (12-week postchemotherapy): no significant change in left orbital lesion on MRI.
- End-of-treatment imaging (24-week postchemotherapy).
  - Orbital MRI: persistent, enhancing, residual left orbit mass (Fig. 9.2).
  - PET/CT: orbital lesion does not demonstrate hypermetabolic activity; no evidence of local regional recurrence or distant metastasis.
- Treatment:
  - Eye-sparing total resection of the residual left orbital mass.
  - Histopathologic analysis of the surgical specimen: embryonal rhabdomyosarcoma with partial treatment effect.
  - Postop MRI: no sign of gross disease.
- Continued maintenance chemotherapy VTC (vinorelbine/temsirolimus/cyclophosphamide) for additional 14 months.

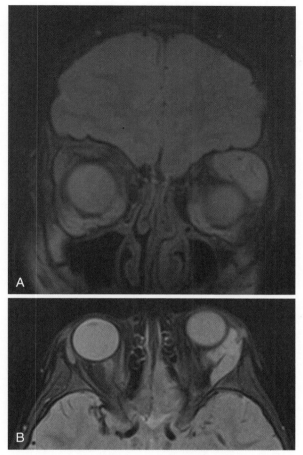

Fig. 9.1 Initial presentation MRI (at another hospital). (A) Coronal and (B) axial orbital MRIs reveal large mass in the left superolateral orbit.

FOLLOW-UP

- Patient remained stable and tumor-free (clinically and radiologically) for 21 months after surgery.
- Recommended continued long-term follow-up for at least 5 years for cancer surveillance in the orbit or elsewhere and also to evaluate for treatment-related ocular side effects (e.g., cataract, dry eye, radiation retinopathy, and orbital hypoplasia).

KEY POINTS

- Rhabdomyosarcoma is the most common primary malignant orbital tumor in children.
- There are two major histologic subtypes, embryonal and alveolar, of which the former is much more common and the latter is more aggressive.
- Diagnosis is done by surgical biopsy, incisional/excisional, depending on the size of tumor and involvement of vital orbital structures.
- Treatment consists of combination chemotherapy and radiotherapy for local control.

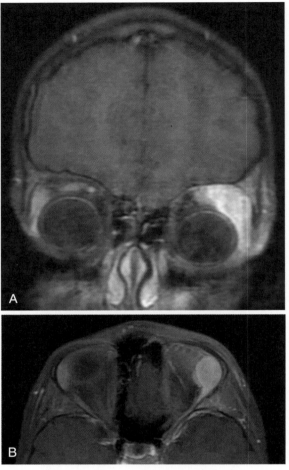

Fig. 9.2 Orbital MRI at the time of presentation; 2 weeks after completing 24 weeks of chemotherapy and radiation therapy, (A) Coronal and (B) axial orbital MRIs demonstrate a residual mass in left superolateral orbit.

- Current chemoradiation protocols are based on the clinical trials of the Intergroup Rhabdomyosarcoma Study Group (IRSG).[1,2]
- A residual orbital mass may be seen on imaging studies at the conclusion of chemoradiation treatment in approximately one-third of patients. The majority of such lesions will either resolve spontaneously or remain stable. The decision whether to re-biopsy should be made on a case-by-case basis.
- Radiologic response at 12 weeks is predictive of long-term outcome, meaning the patients who have minimal response after 12 weeks of chemotherapy have a significantly higher risk of progression.
- Prognosis depends largely on tumor morphology: embryonal cell type is expected to have a 94% 5-year survival rate, while alveolar only has a 74% 5-year survival rate.
- Long-term treatment-related ocular complications include cataract, dry eye, orbital hypoplasia, radiation retinopathy, blepharoptosis, and, rarely, secondary malignancy.

References

1. Crist WM, Anderson JR, Meza JL, et al. Intergroup Rhabdomyosarcoma Study-IV: Results for patients with nonmetastatic disease. *J Clin Oncol*. 2001;19(12):3091–3102. doi:10.1200/JCO.2001.19.12.3091.
2. Crist W, Gehan EA, Ragab AH, et al. The Third Intergroup Rhabdomyosarcoma Study. *J Clin Oncol*. 1995;13(3):610–630. doi:10.1200/JCO.1995.13.3.610.

CHAPTER 10

Orbit Lacrimal Pleomorphic Adenoma

Sang H. Hong

Progressive Unilateral Ptosis in an 11-Year-Old Child

HISTORY OF PRESENT ILLNESS

A previously healthy 11-year-old male presents with left upper eyelid ptosis, slowly progressive over 1 year. He has no prior ocular history or trauma to either eye.

Exam

	OD	OS
Visual acuity	20/20	20/20
Cycloplegic retinoscopy	Plano	Plano +0.50 × 70
Pupils	Equal, reactive, no APD	Equal, reactive, no APD
EOM	Ortho in all gazes, full ductions OU	Ortho in all gazes, full ductions OU
External exam	Normal	Slight left brow elevation from compensatory frontalis recruitment. Slight fullness over left temporal subbrow area. Slight left hypoglobus. No significant proptosis. Slight reduction to globe retropulsion OS. No tenderness to palpation (Fig. 10.1)
Lids/lashes	Normal	3-mm left upper lid ptosis (with frontalis forced relaxed) with normal levator function (Fig. 10.1)
		Prominent left palpebral lobe of the lacrimal gland visible when the left upper lid was lifted up and everted (Fig. 10.1)
Anterior segment	Normal	Normal
Fundus	Normal	Normal

APD, Afferent pupillary defect; *EOM,* extraocular movement; *IOP,* intraocular pressure; *OD,* oculus dexter (right eye); *OS,* oculus sinister (left eye); *OU,* oculus uterque (both eyes).

QUESTIONS TO ASK

- Does the ptosis vary at all throughout the day?
- Is there any diplopia?

No financial interest is associated with the manuscript. No funding support.

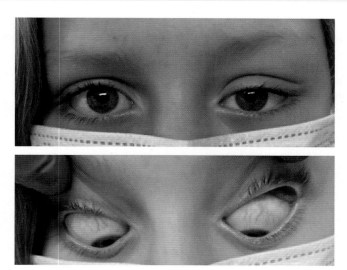

Fig. 10.1 Left upper lid ptosis with left brow elevation from compensatory frontalis recruitment. Fullness over left temporal subbrow area. Prominent left palpebral lobe of the lacrimal gland is visible when the left upper lid was lifted up and everted.

- Is there any vision worsening?
- Does the patient have any pain in or around the left eye, or any pain with eye movement?
- Is there any history of cancer in the family?
- Does the child have any other relevant medical history?

The left upper lid ptosis is constant and not variable. No diplopia in any gaze. Vision is a little blurred in the left eye but overall sees well.

The patient has never complained of pain in or around his left eye. No pain with eye movement. No eye redness. No family history of cancer. No significant past medical history.

ASSESSMENT

- Left upper lid ptosis, likely mechanical.
- Left superotemporal orbital mass possibly involving lacrimal gland.

DIFFERENTIAL DIAGNOSIS

- Lacrimal gland mass
  - Inflammatory (dacryoadenitis): 50% of lacrimal gland masses are inflammatory
    - Idiopathic (nonspecific)
    - Sjögren syndrome
    - Sarcoidosis
    - Antineutrophilic cytoplasmic antibody (ANCA)-associated vasculitis
    - IgG4-related disease
  - Neoplasms
    - Lymphoproliferative (lymphoma, Mikulicz disease): 50% of lacrimal gland neoplasms are lymphoproliferative
    - Epithelial origin

- Benign
  - Pleomorphic adenoma (50% of epithelial tumors are pleomorphic adenomas)
  - Myoepithelioma
  - Oncocytoma
  - Cystadenoma
- Malignant
  - Adenoid cystic carcinoma (50% of lacrimal gland carcinomas are adenoid cystic carcinomas)
  - Adenocarcinoma ex-pleomorphic adenoma
  - Mucoepidermoid carcinoma
  - Squamous carcinoma
- Dermoid
- Dacryops (lacrimal duct cyst)
- Neurofibroma
- Vascular or lymphatic malformation
- Mucocele
- Rhabdomyosarcoma
- Neuroblastoma
- Leukemia

WORKING DIAGNOSIS

- Lymphoma or benign pleomorphic adenoma of lacrimal gland.

INVESTIGATION AND TESTING

- CT: Well-circumscribed, ovoid, likely heterogeneous soft tissue mass in the superolateral aspect of left orbit in extraconal space, displacing lacrimal gland anteriorly and the left superior rectus medially. Left globe is slightly distorted and inferiorly displaced by the mass. Smooth scalloping of superolateral bony orbital wall without osseous destruction or lytic changes, compatible with a slow-growing, nonaggressive tumor (Fig. 10.2).
- MRI: Circumscribed ovoid, heterogeneously T2 hyperintense, T1 isointense, heterogeneously but avidly enhancing mass in extraconal space along superolateral aspect of left globe, causing mild flattening and anteroinferior globe displacement and mild proptosis. Centered in medial half of left lacrimal gland (Fig. 10.3).

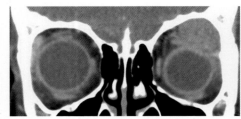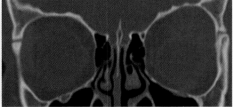

Fig. 10.2 CT of orbits shows a well-circumscribed, ovoid, heterogeneous soft tissue mass in the superolateral aspect of the left orbit in the extraconal space, displacing the lacrimal gland anteriorly and left superior rectus medially. The left globe is slightly distorted and inferiorly displaced by the mass. Smooth scalloping of the superolateral bony orbital wall without osseous destruction or lytic changes is compatible with a slow-growing nonaggressive tumor.

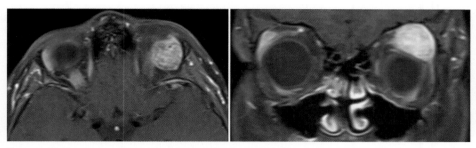

Fig. 10.3 T1 fat-saturated postcontrast MR orbits show a well-circumscribed, heterogeneous, enhancing soft tissue mass in the superolateral aspect of the left orbit extraconal space.

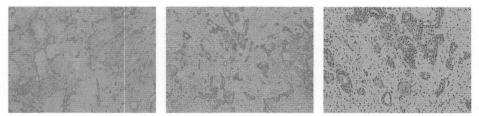

Fig. 10.4 Histopathological examination shows a cellular lesion composed of a mixture of epithelial cells and myoepithelial cells within a background chondromyxoid to fibrous stroma (thus also called *benign mixed tumor*). The tumor cells are arranged in a ductal, tubular, and solid pattern with areas of metaplastic squamous differentiation. The ductal structures are lined by a bilayered cuboidal epithelium. These features are consistent with a cellular pleomorphic adenoma.

MANAGEMENT

- Anterior orbitotomy with total resection of left lacrimal gland mass after a very careful isolated intraoperative incisional frozen-section biopsy (of a well-exposed anterior part of the tumor) confirmed the diagnosis of pleomorphic adenoma (which is more common in older patients [in their fourth and fifth decades] and very rare in the pediatric population). The biopsy site was sealed off with fibrin glue (to prevent any tumor spillage) before the tumor was completely resected. If the clinical diagnosis of pleomorphic adenoma is fairly certain, then the tumor should be resected in its entirety without violating its pseudocapsule, as studies have shown that incomplete excision can lead to recurrence or malignant transformation into adenocarcinoma.
- Histopathology: Relatively circumscribed lesion with peripheral areas of bosselation and nodularity into surrounding capsule but no areas of frank invasion. Lesion is composed of an admixture of epithelial cells predominantly in the form of ducts and tubules with some areas of metaplastic squamous differentiation, myoepithelial cells, and background overall chondromyxoid to fibrous stroma (thus also called *benign mixed tumor*). Also, some areas that are more cellular as well as areas that appear more spindled. Overall features are those of cellular pleomorphic adenoma. No features are worrisome for malignancy, including no significant pleomorphism, mitotic activity (low MIB-1 proliferation rate), or necrosis (Fig. 10.4).

FOLLOW-UP

- The patient did not require any further treatment and has remained stable on follow-up. Plan is to continue to periodically monitor clinically and radiographically for any recurrence.

KEY POINTS

- Pleomorphic adenoma of the lacrimal gland typically presents with slow, insidious, painless, unilateral proptosis, inferomedial displacement of the globe, superotemporal periorbital fullness, and ptosis, usually over the course of a year or more.
- Most commonly presents in the fourth and fifth decades of life and rarely presents in children.
- Radiographic imaging (CT and/or MR orbits) typically will show a soft tissue mass that is solid (but often heterogeneous), well circumscribed, round or ovoid, displacing the globe inferomedially, and sometimes indenting it, with occasional calcifications, and causing smooth scalloping of the superolateral bony orbital wall (lacrimal fossa) without osseous destruction or lytic changes, compatible with a slow-growing, nonaggressive tumor. This is important as distinction to adenoid cystic carcinoma, which usually shows irregular margins, nodularity with infiltration of adjacent tissue, and bony destruction.
- If the clinical impression of pleomorphic adenoma (based on history, exam, and imaging) is very high, then the tumor should be resected in its entirety without violating its pseudocapsule, as studies have shown that incomplete excision can lead to recurrence or malignant transformation into adenocarcinoma. However, if there is diagnostic uncertainty, then a very careful and limited biopsy can be considered, using techniques to avoid any tumor cell spillage.
- The prognosis for these patients is generally favorable if the tumor is completely resected.

CHAPTER 11

Orbit Metastatic Tumor

Komal Bakal ■ Dilip K.R. Mishra ■ Swathi Kaliki

Right Eye Proptosis and Epiphora in a 4-Year-Old Child for 1 Month

HISTORY OF PRESENT ILLNESS

A 4-year-old male child presented with history of forward protrusion (Fig. 11.1) and watering from the right eye. Child had a history of trauma 1 month earlier. There were no other ocular or systemic complaints.

Exam

	OD	OS
External face	Fullness in temporal and zygomatic region	
Ocular position	Proptosis	
	Dystopia; eye was turned inward and upward	
Lymph nodes		Palpable submandibular lymph node
Visual acuity	Can fix and follow light	Can fix and follow light
Anterior segment	Normal	Normal
Posterior segment	Normal	Normal

QUESTIONS TO ASK

- Has the child complained of any headache or eye pain?
- Are there any associated systemic complaints?
- Is there any family history of tumors?

The child did not complain of headache or eye pain. There were no associated systemic symptoms and no family history of tumors.

ASSESSMENT

- Orbital/retroorbital mass involving temporal and zygomatic bone pushing the eyeball outward and nasally
- Possibly a triradiate lesion

No financial interest associated with the manuscript. No funding supports.

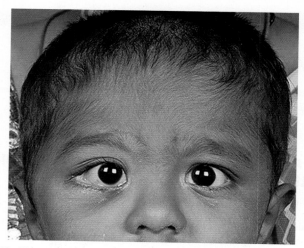

Fig. 11.1   A 4-year-old child presented with proptosis of the right eye.

DIFFERENTIAL DIAGNOSIS

- Rhabdomyosarcoma
- Ewing sarcoma
- Orbital metastasis

WORKING DIAGNOSIS

- Right eye orbital space–occupying lesion

INVESTIGATION AND TESTING

- CT orbit: Ill-defined heterogenous osteolytic lesion involving bilateral orbits, zygomatic and temporal bones (right > left). There was no evidence of intracranial tumor extension (Fig. 11.2).

MANAGEMENT

- The child underwent incisional biopsy of the right orbital lesion along with bone marrow biopsy. Fine-needle aspiration cytology (FNAC) was done from the left submandibular lymph node.
- Histopathology confirmed malignant round cell tumor with involvement of bone marrow. Ki-67 index was high. On immunohistochemical examination, synaptophysin and chromogranin A stains were positive, indicating neuroendocrine tumor (Fig. 11.3). FNAC of the submandibular node was suggestive of granulomatous lymphadenitis.
- Patient was advised of whole-body PET CT, which revealed left suprarenal mass (likely neuroblastoma) with lymph node and multiple skeletal metastases (Fig. 11.4).
- Child was referred to medical oncologist for further management.

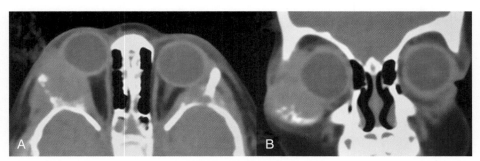

Fig. 11.2 CT orbit (A) axial and (B) coronal sections showing ill-defined, heterogenous extraconal lesions in bilateral orbit with adjacent bone erosion.

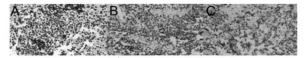

Fig. 11.3 Histopathology showing (A) singly scattered and loose clusters of small round cells (H&E stain; 40x maginification), (B) membranous synoptophysisn positivity (immune stain; 40x magnification), (C) chromogranin A positivity (immune stain; 40x magnification).

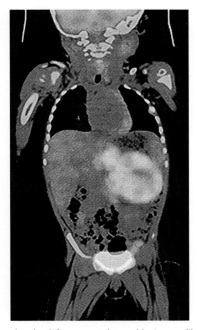

Fig. 11.4 Whole-body PET scan showing left suprarenal neuroblastoma with multiple skeletal metastasis.

FOLLOW-UP

- Undergoing palliative care

KEY POINTS

- Orbital metastases comprise 1% to 13% of all orbital neoplasms, and the incidence of orbital metastases in patients with systemic malignancy is 2% to 5%.
- In adults, the most common primary tumors to metastasize to orbit are neoplasms of the breast, prostate, lung, kidney, and gastrointestinal tract.
- Orbital metastases in children are rare, and the most common tumor to metastasize to the orbit is adrenal neuroblastoma. Others include Wilms tumor and Ewing sarcoma.
- Whole-body PET CT is recommended in cases with suspicion of metastasis but with no known history of primary tumor.
- Surgical resection of the tumor/debulking followed by chemotherapy or radiotherapy as appropriate should be performed in consultation with a medical oncologist.
- In cases of unresectable tumors, incisional biopsy followed by chemotherapy and/or radiotherapy as appropriate are employed.
- The prognosis of patients with orbital metastases is poor, with 1-year survival rate of 40%.

CHAPTER 12

Orbit Lacrimal Adenoid Cystic Carcinoma

Komal Bakal ▦ Saumya Jakati ▦ Swathi Kaliki

Proptosis and Pain in a 32-Year-Old Female

HISTORY OF PRESENT ILLNESS

A 32-year-old female presented with complaints of right eye proptosis (Fig. 12.1) for 1 year. There was no history of trauma or thyroid dysfunction.

Exam

	OD	OS
Ocular position	Axial proptosis of 4 mm	Normal
Extraocular movements	Full and free	Full and free
Palpation	Firm tender mass in superotemporal orbit	
Lymph node examination	No regional lymphadenopathy	
Visual acuity	20/20	20/20
IOP (mm Hg)	15	15
Sclera/conjunctiva	White and quiet	White and quiet
Cornea	Clear	Clear
AC	Deep and quiet	Deep and quiet
Iris	Unremarkable	Unremarkable
Lens	Clear	Clear
Anterior vitreous	Clear	Clear
Retina/optic nerve	Normal	Normal

AC, Anterior chamber; *IOP,* intraocular pressure.

QUESTIONS TO ASK

- Do you experience pain?
- Have you experienced any systemic complaints?

Patient was experiencing pain in the right periocular area with associated right-sided headache for 1 year. There were no other systemic complaints.

ASSESSMENT

- Abaxial proptosis.
- Orbital space-occupying lesion mostly arising from the right lacrimal gland.

No financial interest is associated with the manuscript. No funding support.

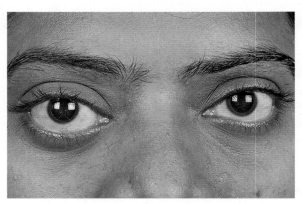

Fig. 12.1   A 32-year-old female with proptosis of the right eye.

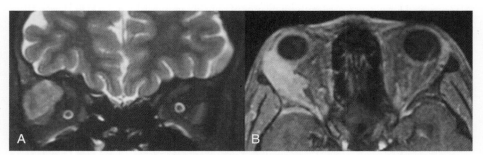

Fig. 12.2   MRI orbit revealing (A) well-defined heterogenous hyperintense lacrimal gland lesion in the right orbit with (B) contrast enhancement.

DIFFERENTIAL DIAGNOSIS

- Pleomorphic adenoma
- Adenoid cystic carcinoma
- Lacrimal gland adenocarcinoma

WORKING DIAGNOSIS

- Right lacrimal gland adenoid cystic carcinoma.

INVESTIGATION AND TESTING

- MRI orbit: Right eye proptosis with well-defined heterogenous hyperintense infiltrative lacrimal gland lesion (Fig. 12.2A) with contrast enhancement (Fig. 12.2B) extending until the midorbit. Lateral rectus muscle was indistinct from the mass until the midorbit.

MANAGEMENT

- Patient underwent excisional biopsy of the right lacrimal gland lesion, which was removed en bloc via lateral orbitotomy followed by external beam radiotherapy (EBRT).

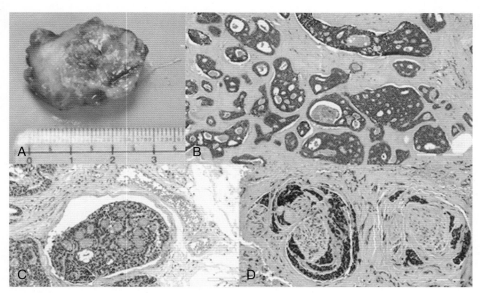

Fig. 12.3 (A) Gross specimen of the excised mass showing irregular solid mass measuring 3 cm × 2 cm in size. Photomicrographs showing (B) tumor predominantly arranged in cribriform (Swiss cheese–like) pattern with background hyalinization (hematoxylin and eosin [H&E] staining; original magnification, 14x) with (C) intra-lesional vascular embolus (H&E staining; original magnification, 30x) and (D) perineural invasion (H&E staining; original magnification, 30x).

- Histopathology revealed adenoid cystic carcinoma of lacrimal gland with perineural invasion and vascular emboli (Figs. 12.3A–D).
- Patient underwent whole body PET CT, which showed no evidence of systemic metastasis.

FOLLOW-UP

- The patient did not require any further treatment and is currently in remission.

KEY POINTS

- Although a rare tumor, adenoid cystic carcinoma is the most common malignant epithelial tumor of the lacrimal gland.
- Pain is a cardinal symptom, caused by perineural invasion.
- Adenoid cystic carcinoma is an aggressive tumor due to its tendency for perineural invasion, spread along the periosteal planes, and high chances of recurrence. Prognosis is poor with less than 50% survival rate at 5 years and less than 20% at 10 years.
- Prognosis depends on various factors such as histopathological variant, age, perineural invasion, tumor stage, and presence of apoptotic factors.
- Current treatment strategy includes eye-sparing surgical resection wherever possible or orbital exenteration followed by adjuvant EBRT.
- Area for radiation should include surgical area with 5-mm margin surrounding it, along with lateral orbital wall, superior orbital fissure, orbital roof, and nerve tract up to the skull base.
- Other adjuvant therapies include proton beam therapy and intensity-modulated radiotherapy.

CHAPTER 13

Optic Nerve Pilocytic Astrocytoma (Glioma)

Elizabeth Miller Bolton ■ Janice Lasky Zeid

11-Month Old Male With Multiple Café Au Lait Spots

HISTORY OF PRESENT ILLNESS

An 11-month-old male presents to the ophthalmology clinic, referred by his pediatrician for an exam on the basis of multiple café au lait spots and suspicion of neurofibromatosis type 1 (NF1). Patient had multiple café au lait spots first noted at 4 months of age. Family history was negative for NF or café au lait spots. By history, no vision concerns and eyes tracking well.

At initial exam, the patient had no ocular manifestations of NF1. Vision acuity (VA) was normal for age 20/94 each eye using Teller acuity cards. Bilateral anterior segment exam was unremarkable with no iris Lisch nodules, and dilated exam revealed normal optic nerve appearance each eye with C:D 0.1. Diagnosis of NF1 was not made at that time as findings were limited to café au lait spots.

On follow-up at age 2 years, the patient had developed inguinal freckling. Based on this second criteria, a diagnosis of NF1 was made. Parents had no visual concerns.

Patient monitored yearly with a stable exam until he presented at 5 years old with 3-mm proptosis of his right eye.

Exam

	Age: 5 Years	
	OD	**OS**
Visual acuity	20/20 (HOTV)	20/20 (HOTV)
IOP (mm Hg)	20	9
Sclera/conjunctiva	White and quiet	White and quiet
Cornea	Clear	Clear
AC	Deep and quiet	Deep and quiet
Iris	No Lisch nodules	+ Lisch nodules
Lens	Clear	Clear
Anterior vitreous	Normal, no cells	Normal, no cells
Retina/optic nerve	3+ edema, no pallor, no disc hemorrhages (Fig. 13.3)	No edema, no disc hemorrhages, no pallor (Fig. 13.3)

AC, Anterior chamber; *IOP,* intraocular pressure.

No financial interest associated with the manuscript. No funding supports.

At an exam at age 5 years, VA remained 20/20 in each eye via HOTV optotypes. Color vision was 5/6 using Hardy-Rand-Rittler in each eye. Exophthalmometry revealed 3-mm proptosis right eye. Iris Lisch nodules were noted in the left eye. Dilated exam revealed right optic nerve 3+ elevation, no pallor or disc hemorrhages, and unremarkable left optic nerve.

QUESTIONS TO ASK

- Any family history of NF1?
- Relevant past medical history or birth history?
- Any skin findings (e.g., café au lait spots)?
- Any other neurologic symptoms or tumors?
- Complaint of decreased vision or vision changes?
- Any episodes of eye pain?

This patient had no family history of NF1 and initially had café au lait spots as an isolated finding. NF1 was later diagnosed with second criteria of freckling. Birth history was unremarkable, and the patient had no other medical history outside of NF1. Patient had no vision changes. He developed proptosis but had no eye pain and no history of neurologic symptoms or known tumors.

ASSESSMENT

- NF1
- Lisch nodules
- Proptosis right eye
- 3+ disc edema right eye

DIFFERENTIAL DIAGNOSIS

- Optic pathway glioma
- Orbital plexiform neurofibroma
- Lymphoma
- Inflammatory pseudotumor
- Inflammatory disorder of optic nerve (i.e., optic neuritis)
- Increased intracranial pressure

WORKING DIAGNOSIS

- Optic pathway glioma associated with NF1 (OPG-NF1)

INVESTIGATION AND TESTING

- MRI performed due to proptosis and optic elevation. Right eye revealed fusiform enlargement of the intraorbital segment of the right optic nerve with restricted diffusion and avid enhancement consistent with optic pathway glioma (Fig. 13.1).
- Genetic testing showed *NF1* c.2887C>T (p.Gln963Ter), a nonsense variant causing premature stop codon.

MANAGEMENT

- Initial close follow-up: stable with eye exams every 4–6 weeks.
- Repeat MRI brain/orbits 3 months after initial MRI showed no progression of OPG.

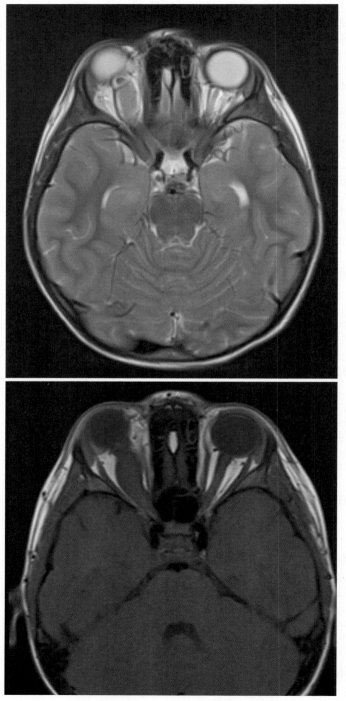

Fig. 13.1 MRI brain and orbits axial images: axial T2 blade *(above)*, axial T1 *(below)*.

- Progression of symptoms 6 months after diagnosis of OPG-NF1: VA right eye decreased to 20/25, left eye 20/20 via Snellen chart, worsening proptosis (by 1 mm–2 mm) right eye, and repeat MRI showed mild progression of OPG.
- Decision to treat: given progression of symptoms (proptosis, decreased vision) and progression of OPG-NF1 on imaging, chemotherapy was initiated to prevent further vision loss and proptosis that might lead to exposure. Carboplatin/vincristine chemotherapy 1-year course: improvement in optic disc edema right eye (trace elevation remaining and mild temporal pallor) and improvement of proptosis (by 1 mm–2 mm). Patient completed 1 year of chemotherapy and continued to have frequent ophthalmology follow-up. After completion of chemotherapy, VA in the right eye was stable at 20/20-3 and left eye 20/20. His color vision was 5/6 in the right eye and 6/6 in the left eye. Proptosis and optic nerve appearance remained stable (Fig. 13.2).

FOLLOW-UP

- During chemotherapy treatment: follow-up exam every 3 months stable.
- After chemotherapy completed: follow-up exam every 6 months, and patient has remained stable for 2 years. Currently monitored with MRI brain and orbits every 6 months. At around age 6, he was also monitored with ocular coherence tomography (OCT) measuring peripapillary retinal nerve fiber layer (RNFL) thickness, which remained stable over time.

KEY POINTS

- Neurofibromatosis type 1 (NF1) is an autosomal dominant genetic disease.
- Approximately 95% of NF1 patients meet diagnostic criteria by age 8 years, and all meet criteria by age 20 years (see diagnostic criteria in Table 13.1).
- OPGs are low-grade astrocytomas and occur in approximately 15–20% of NF1 patients, typically presenting prior to age 6 years, although symptomatic tumors have been reported in older children.
- Visual deterioration is often the first presenting sign of OPG, and therefore VA testing at ophthalmology exams is critical to following patients with OPG.
- OPG-NF1 has a benign course in many cases, with approximately one-half to two-thirds of patients having minimal tumor progression. One-third to one-half of OPGs cause significant morbidity, including vision loss, disfiguring proptosis, and endocrine abnormalities.
- Sporadic OPGs (not associated with NF1) progress more frequently and have a worse prognosis.
- Decision to treat is a challenge: some advocate to treat with either radiographic progression or visual deterioration, whereas others reserve treatment only for OPG with documented visual deterioration. Clinical behavior of OPG varies significantly; however, the presence of symptoms at diagnosis, occurring in about 60% of patients, is the best predictor of the need for treatment. Tumor location does convey outcome, as more posterior visual pathway OPGs are more likely to progress. Tumor size/extent, location, progressive proptosis, optic pallor, and visual field loss are all factors to consider (Fig. 13.3).
- Currently, chemotherapy is the first-line treatment for OPG in most ophthalmology centers. Standard treatment includes a combination of vincristine and carboplatin that has been effective in controlling progressive and recurrent OPGs. Alternatively, vinblastine may be used if hypersensitivity is present or as initial treatment. There is ongoing study of selumetinib, a mitogen-activated extracellular signal-regulated kinase (MEK) inhibitor, in comparison with standard treatment for patients with OPG-NF1.
- Radiotherapy is no longer commonly used for the treatment of OPG due to adverse side effects, including cognitive, vision, and life-threatening complications, as well as risk for secondary tumors.

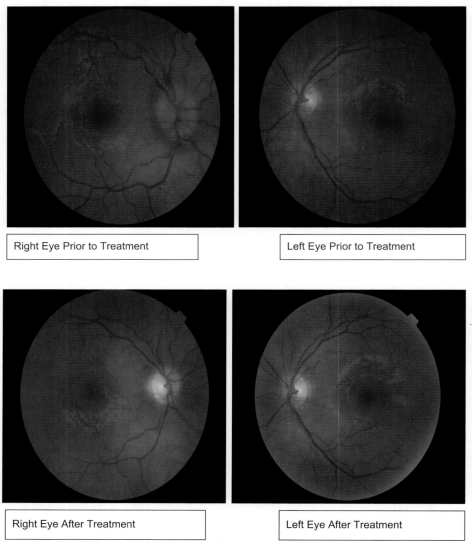

Right Eye Prior to Treatment

Left Eye Prior to Treatment

Right Eye After Treatment

Left Eye After Treatment

Fig. 13.2 Fundus photography of right eye and left eye upon new onset of right eye proptosis, optic disc edema *(above)*, and 1 year after treatment with chemotherapy *(below)*.

- Surgery is rarely indicated for OPG, and surgical biopsy is not indicated except for cases with unusual clinical or radiographic features; surgery is reserved for painful or disfiguring proptosis, corneal exposure, or blind painful eye.
- Optical coherence tomography (OCT) is a newer modality to aid monitoring children with OPG, studied in children age 6 years and older. Peripapillary RNFL thickness was found to be decreased in most children who had abnormal VA or a visual field defect. It is another helpful parameter to use in monitoring OPG-NF1.

TABLE 13.1 ■ Diagnostic Criteria for Neurofibromatosis Type 1 (NF1)

At least two of the criteria listed in the table must be present for diagnosis of NF1.
Six or more café au lait spots over 5 mm in greatest diameter in prepubertal individuals and over 15 mm in greatest diameter in postpubertal individuals
Two or more neurofibromas or one plexiform neurofibroma
Axillary or inguinal freckling
Optic pathway glioma
Two or more iris Lisch nodules or two or more choroidal abnormalities: bright patchy nodules on OCT/ near-infrared reflectance (NIR) imaging
Characteristic skeletal dysplasia (sphenoid wing dysplasia, long-bone dysplasia)
An affected first-degree relative diagnosed by the above criteria
A pathogenic NF1 gene variant

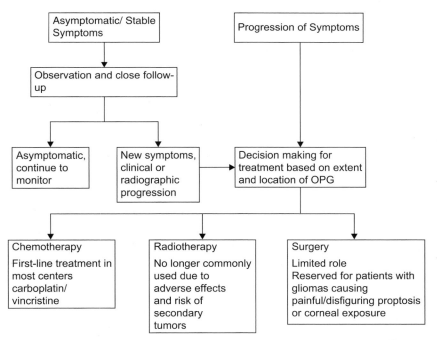

Fig. 13.3 Decision-making pathway in considering treatment for optic pathway gliomas (OPGs).

CHAPTER 14

Optic Nerve Sheath Meningioma

Abigail Jebaraj ■ Judith Warner ■ Sravanthi Vegunta

Decreased Unilateral Visual Acuity in a 12-Year-Old Female

HISTORY OF PRESENT ILLNESS

A previously healthy 12-year-old female presents with decreased visual acuity in the left eye, worsening over 2 years. She has noted difficulty seeing the board at school and relies on her right eye to see. She has no prior ocular history or trauma to either eye.

Exam

	OD	OS
Visual acuity (with correction)	20/20	20/125
Sclera/conjunctiva	White and quiet	White and quiet
Cornea	Clear	Clear
AC	Deep and quiet	Deep and quiet
Iris	Round and reactive, no lesions on iris	Round and reactive, no lesions on iris, 1.8 log units afferent pupillary defect
Lens	Clear	Clear
Anterior vitreous	Clear	Clear
Retina/optic nerve	Normal optic nerve, posterior and peripheral retina (Fig. 14.1A)	Pallor of left optic nerve with normal posterior pole and peripheral retina (Fig.14.1B)

AC, Anterior chamber.

Additional testing: Color vision is normal on the right and control only on the left. Stereopsis is absent. On Hertel exophthalmometry, she has 2 mm of left-sided proptosis. Flicker fusion testing demonstrates reduced function in the left eye compared to the right. Her Humphrey visual field 24-2 testing of the right eye is normal, while the left eye demonstrates a dense nasal hemianopia with central scotoma (Fig. 14.2). Her optical coherence tomography of the retinal nerve fiber layer (OCT RNFL) reveals only borderline temporal thinning of the left optic nerve (Fig. 14.3).

No financial interest is associated with the manuscript. No funding support.

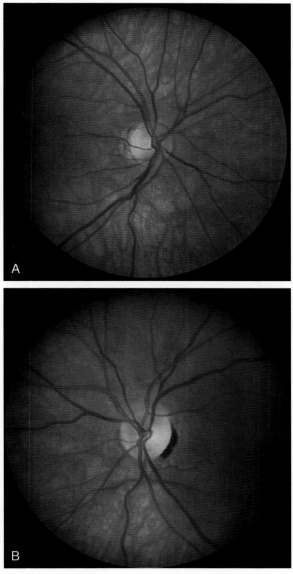

Fig. 14.1   (A) Normal right optic nerve and vessels. (B) Left optic nerve with temporal pallor, peripapillary pigment, and normal vessels.

QUESTIONS TO ASK

- Has your daughter ever had redness or pain in her left eye?
- Is there any history of cancers or tumors in the family?
- Does she have any other relevant past medical history?

The patient has never complained of pain in her left eye. There has been no eye redness bilaterally. There is no family history of cancer. Her parents deny any other significant past medical history.

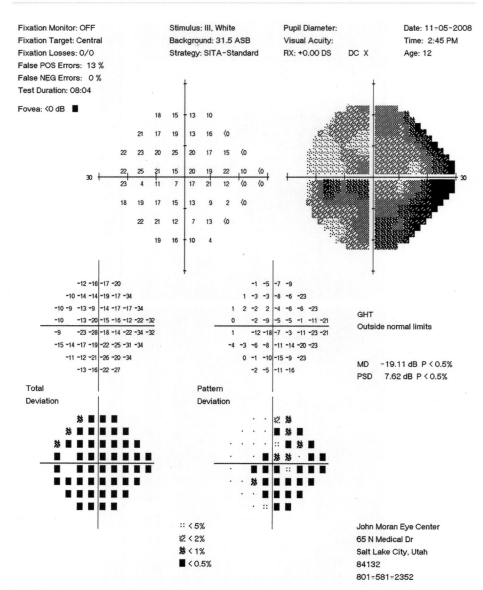

Fig. 14.2 Humphrey visual field 24-2 of the left eye demonstrates dense nasal hemianopia with central scotoma. Mean deviation was −19.11. Pattern standard deviation was 7.62 dB.

ASSESSMENT

- Painless left optic nerve atrophy with mild proptosis in a child.

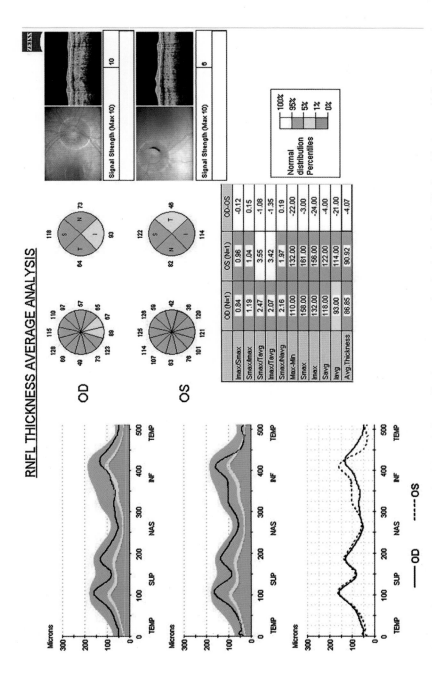

Fig. 14.3 Optical coherence tomography of the retinal nerve fiber layer at presentation showing borderline thinning of the temporal left optic nerve at 46 μm. The average thickness of the right nerve was 87 μm, and the left nerve was 91 μm.

DIFFERENTIAL DIAGNOSIS

- Optic nerve glioma
- Optic nerve sheath meningioma
- Metastatic disease of the orbit
- Leukemic infiltration of the optic nerve
- Neurosarcoidosis
- Tuberculosis
- Optic perineuritis
- Myelin oligodendrocytic glycoprotein (MOG) optic neuritis
- Traumatic optic neuropathy
- Congenital optic nerve atrophy

WORKING DIAGNOSIS

- Optic nerve sheath mass, left eye.

INVESTIGATION AND TESTING

- MRI Brain: 1.8 cm (anterior–posterior) × 1.1 cm (transverse) × 1.2 cm (craniocaudally) solid enhancing mass arising from the left optic nerve. The mass was isointense on T1 without gadolinium and hyperintense on T2. The mass involved the intraorbital portion of the optic nerve without extending into the chiasm or hypothalamus (Fig. 14.4).

MANAGEMENT

- The patient underwent a biopsy of the left optic nerve mass to determine if the mass was an optic nerve glioma or an optic nerve sheath meningioma.
- Pathology was positive for a World Health Organization (WHO) grade I meningioma.
- At 1 month after initial presentation, the patient's vision had worsened to 20/400 with a 2.4-log unit left relative afferent pupillary defect and 3 mm of left-sided proptosis. Her fundus examination showed left optic nerve pallor and new retinal striae. Repeat imaging did not show a significant change in the size of the mass. However, she was encouraged to proceed with the treatment due to the vision changes.
- After discussing options of radiation therapy, chemotherapy, or surgery, she and her parents elected for radiation therapy. She received conventional fractionated radiotherapy and received a total dose of 54 Gy in 39 fractions. Her vision improved to 20/20 after radiation therapy. She also recovered stereopsis and color vision. Her left eye proptosis decreased to 1 mm. Her left relative afferent pupillary defect decreased to 0.6 log units.

FOLLOW-UP

- At her most recent follow-up 15 years after initial presentation, the patient's visual acuity and testing were stable. MRI brain showed no interval changes and no new meningiomas elsewhere (Fig. 14.5). Her left eye visual acuity was 20/20. She had a 0.6 log unit afferent pupillary defect. Her left optic nerve on exam was pale (Fig. 14.6), and her OCT RNFL demonstrated stable atrophy from prior years (Fig. 14.7). Her Humphrey visual field 24-2 testing of the left eye demonstrated only a few scattered inferior defects with recovery of the majority of her visual field (Fig. 14.8).

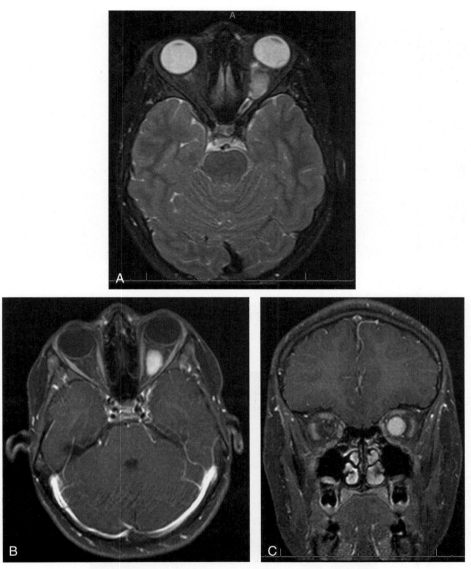

Fig. 14.4 (A) MRI brain T2 axial fat-saturated image at initial presentation of the left optic nerve lesion showing hyperintense mass, posterior globe compression, and proptosis. The lesion is 1.8 cm (anterior–posterior) x 1.1 cm (transverse) x 1.2 cm (craniocaudally). (B) T1 postcontrast axial fat-saturated image at initial presentation shows homogeneous enhancement of the left optic nerve lesion. (C) T1 postcontrast fat-saturated coronal view of the left optic nerve lesion again shows diffuse enhancement of the lesion.

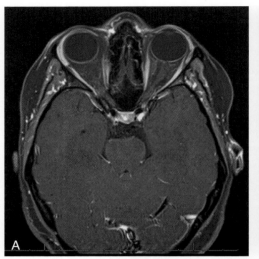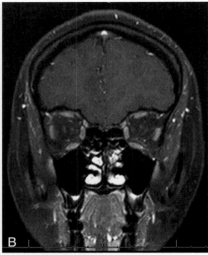

Fig. 14.5 (A) T1 postcontrast axial fat-saturated image at 10-year follow-up shows decrease in size of left optic nerve lesion and no enhancement. (B) T1 postcontrast fat-saturated coronal view of the left optic nerve showing resolution of lesion and no enhancement at 10-year follow-up.

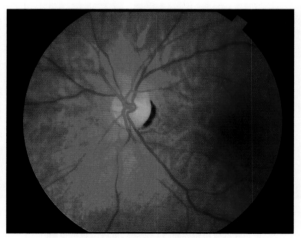

Fig. 14.6 Left optic nerve with stable temporal pallor, peripapillary pigment, and normal vessels 15 years after presentation.

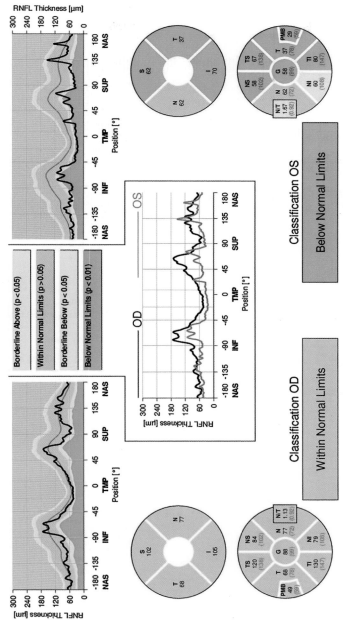

Fig. 14.7 Optical coherence tomography of the retinal nerve fiber layer of both eyes 15 years after initial presentation, and after radiation therapy of the left optic nerve. Right optic nerve is of normal thickness with average thickness of 87 μm. Left eye shows superior, inferior, and temporal thinning of the left optic nerve with average thickness of 58 μm. The left optic nerve thinning has remained stable for several years following radiation.

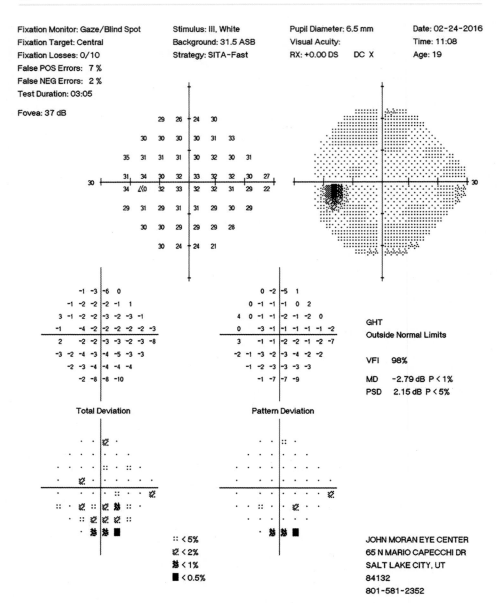

Fixation Monitor: Gaze/Blind Spot
Fixation Target: Central
Fixation Losses: 0/10
False POS Errors: 7 %
False NEG Errors: 2 %
Test Duration: 03:05

Fovea: 37 dB

Stimulus: III, White
Background: 31.5 ASB
Strategy: SITA-Fast

Pupil Diameter: 6.5 mm
Visual Acuity:
RX: +0.00 DS   DC X

Date: 02-24-2016
Time: 11:08
Age: 19

GHT
Outside Normal Limits

VFI   98%

MD   -2.79 dB P < 1%
PSD   2.15 dB P < 5%

Total Deviation

Pattern Deviation

:: < 5%
⌧ < 2%
⧆ < 1%
■ < 0.5%

JOHN MORAN EYE CENTER
65 N MARIO CAPECCHI DR
SALT LAKE CITY, UT
84132
801-581-2352

Fig. 14.8 Humphrey Visual Field 24-2 of the left eye 8 years after presentation and following radiation therapy shows a recovery of peripheral vision with only a few scattered inferior defects remaining. Mean deviation is –2.79; pattern standard deviation is 2.15 dB; visual field index is 98%.

KEY POINTS

- Optic nerve sheath meningiomas (ONSMs) arise from meningoepithelial cell proliferation of the arachnoid villi of the optic nerve sheath.
- They account for 1–2% of all meningiomas, 10% of orbital meningiomas, and 33% of primary optic nerve tumors.
- 95% of ONSMs are unilateral and are most often diagnosed in women at a mean age of 60 years. They are rare in children but can be more aggressive with more rapid progression and significant vision loss. ONSMs in children have been associated with neurofibromatosis type 2 (NF2).
- Optic pathway gliomas are more common in children than ONSMs and can present in 15–20% of children with neurofibromatosis type 1 (NF1). Optic pathway gliomas are also typically less aggressive than childhood ONSMs.
- Typical presenting symptoms and signs of ONSM include painless, slowly progressive vision loss in one eye, optic nerve edema and/or atrophy, optociliary shunt vessels, relative afferent pupillary defect, visual field changes, proptosis, and extraocular motility deficits.
- Stereotactic fractionated radiation therapy is the mainstay of treatment if warranted. If there are no significant visual effects, ONSMs can be observed closely. Side effects of radiation are rare and can include radiation retinopathy, optic neuropathy, central retinal artery occlusion, and pituitary dysfunction. Other treatment options are surgical resection, particularly if there is intracranial extension, but there is a higher risk of vision loss.

Conjunctival Tumors

CHAPTER 15

Conjunctival Lipodermoid

Azza M.Y. Maktabi ■ Rawan Althaqib

Conjunctival Mass in a 12-Year-Old Female

HISTORY OF PRESENT ILLNESS

A 12-year-old female presents with a temporal large pinkish-yellow mass in her left eye since birth, not changing in size (Fig. 15.1). Excision was attempted by local ophthalmologist 1 year earlier. Otherwise, she is a healthy girl with no history of previous trauma.

Exam

	OD	OS
Visual acuity	20/20	20/20
Eyelids and external	Normal	Fullness of the lateral canthus
Sclera/conjunctiva	White and quiet	Lateral canthus large pinkish-yellow conjunctival immobile mass is noted extending temporally up to the upper and lower fornices, while the temporal margin cannot be traced; few hair shafts noted on the surface
Cornea	Clear	Clear
AC	Deep and quiet	Deep and quiet
Iris	Unremarkable	Unremarkable
Lens	Clear	Clear
Retina/optic nerve	Normal optic nerve, posterior and peripheral retina	Normal optic nerve, posterior and peripheral retina

AC, Anterior chamber.

QUESTIONS TO ASK

- Has this mass increased in size?
- Does the mass affect the vision?
- Have you had any other systemic illnesses?

The patient has never complained of pain in her eye or change in vision. The mass is slowly increasing in size. There are no signs of redness in both eyes. There is no history of cancer in the family. Parents deny any other significant past medical history.

No financial interest associated with the manuscript. No funding supports.

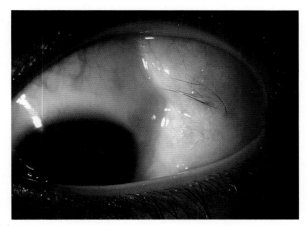

Fig. 15.1 Left eye showing a pinkish-yellow mass temporally. Hair shafts are noted.

ASSESSMENT

Lateral canthus large yellow conjunctival immobile mass is noted extending temporally up to the upper and lower fornices, extension posteriorly into the orbit. Few hair shafts are noted on the surface. No periauricular skin appendages.

DIFFERENTIAL DIAGNOSIS

- Lipodermoid
- Herniated orbital fat
- Neoplasm of the lacrimal gland
- Lacrimal gland prolapse

WORKING DIAGNOSIS

- Conjunctival lipodermoid (dermolipoma), OS

INVESTIGATION AND TESTING

- MRI of brain and orbits: Well-circumscribed mass seen along the left orbit that appears as a fat-containing lesion measuring 21.1 mm × 7.9 mm in diameter, seen at the lacrimal gland bed. No evidence of mass effect or deeper extension. No evidence of abnormal enhancement following intravenous injection of contrast media. No evidence of surrounding inflammatory changes.

MANAGEMENT

- Patient underwent excision of the mass of OS.
- Histopathology revealed a mass lined by keratinized stratified squamous epithelium with skin appendages. The subepithelial tissue was composed of dense collagen fibers typically seen in dermoid cysts, with a large area of adipose tissue (Fig. 15.2).

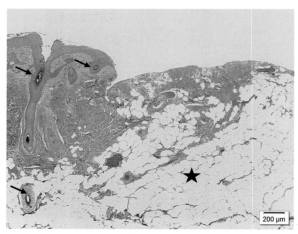

Fig. 15.2 The conjunctival mass is lined by keratinized epithelium with hair follicles *(arrow)* surrounded by dense stroma. A large area of the mass is composed of mature adipose tissue *(star)*.

FOLLOW-UP

- The patient was seen postoperatively and has a well-healed scar.

KEY POINTS

- Conjunctival lipodermoid is a benign lesion; though congenital, it could be clinically noticeable in the first decade of life.
- Commonly found in the superotemporal quadrant as a yellow immobile mass.
- Management is observation unless it is cosmetically intolerable, in which case excision is advised.
- Could be missed as herniated orbital fat, which is usually bilateral, mobile, possibly retractable, and more fatty yellow in color.
- Lipodermoid could be part of systemic manifestation of Goldenhar syndrome or organoid nevus syndrome.

Conjunctival Nevus

Jaxon Huang ▪ Elyana Vittoria Tessa Locatelli ▪ Carol Karp ▪ Anat Galor

65-Year-Old With Pigmented Conjunctival Lesion

HISTORY OF PRESENT ILLNESS

- The patient reports visual distortions in the left eye and notes that the pigmented lesion has been present for years.
- The patient also has a past history of bone marrow cancer.

Exam

	OD	OS
Visual acuity	20/40-1	20/40-2
IOP (mm Hg)	15	14
Conjunctiva/sclera	White and quiet	Brown, pigmented, cystic lesion at 10:00 superior to nasal pterygium
Cornea	Clear	Pterygium at 9:00 with adjacent area of opalescence at 6:00–7:00 (Fig. 16.1)
AC	Deep and quiet	Deep and quiet
Iris	Unremarkable	Unremarkable
	Brown iris, pupil round, no NVI	Brown iris, pupil round, no NVI
Lens	1+ nuclear sclerosis	1+ nuclear sclerosis
Anterior vitreous	Clear	Clear
Retina/optic nerve	Normal optic nerve, posterior and peripheral retina	Normal optic nerve, posterior and peripheral retina

AC, Anterior chamber; *IOP,* intraocular pressure; *NVI,* neovascularization of the iris.

QUESTIONS TO ASK

- Around what age did you first notice the pigmented lesion? Has it been there your entire life?
- Have you noticed any changes in the size or color of the pigmented lesion?

No financial interest associated with the manuscript.

Supported by the Department of Veterans Affairs, Veterans Health Administration, Office of Research and Development, Clinical Sciences R&D (CSRD) I01 CX002015 (Dr. Galor), Biomedical Laboratory R&D (BLRD) Service I01 BX004893 (Dr. Galor), Rehabilitation R&D (RRD) I21 RX003883 (Dr. Galor); Department of Defense Gulf War Illness Research Program (GWIRP) W81XWH-20-1-0579 (Dr. Galor) and Vision Research Program (VRP) W81XWH-20-1-0820 (Dr. Galor); National Eye Institute U01 EY034686 (Dr. Galor), U24EY035102 (Dr. Galor), R33EY032468 (Dr. Galor); and NIH Center Core Grant P30EY014801 (institutional) and Research to Prevent Blindness Unrestricted Grant GR004596-1 (institutional).

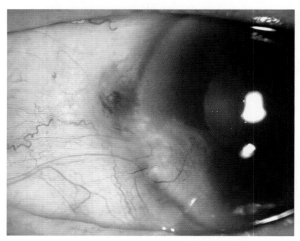

Fig. 16.1 Slit lamp photo of a pigmented, slightly elevated, cystic appearing lesion located at 10:00 in the left eye.

- Do you have any irritation or pain in the left eye?
- Have you ever seen an optometrist or ophthalmologist for the pigmented lesion, and if so, were pictures of it taken?

The patient has noted the pigmented lesion for many years and has not noticed any changes. There are no documented images of the lesion, and she has no symptoms in her eye.

ASSESSMENT

- Given the long-standing presence, cystic-appearing components, and location in the nasal quadrant of the interpalpebral bulbar conjunctiva, the lesion may be a benign conjunctival nevus (CN).
- However, given that the lesion is noncircumscribed, crosses the limbus, and extends onto the cornea, and the fact that CN has the ability to transform into malignant melanoma, malignancy cannot be ruled out based on clinical examination alone.

DIFFERENTIAL DIAGNOSIS

- The differential diagnosis of pigmented conjunctival lesions includes CN, primary acquired melanosis (PAM), complexion-associated melanosis (CAM), malignant melanoma (MM), and ocular melanocytosis.
- CN are benign, well-circumscribed, variably elevated, and variably pigmented lesions with clear cysts scattered within the pigment. They are most commonly located in the interpalpebral bulbar conjunctiva in either the temporal or nasal quadrants.
- PAM primarily occurs in white individuals as a pigmented, flat, noncircumscribed, unilateral lesion that lacks cystic components. PAM can either be benign (PAM without atypia) or have a chance of malignant transformation (PAM with atypia).
- CAM primarily occurs in darkly pigmented individuals as a diffuse, flat, noncircumscribed, patchy, pigmented lesion located near the limbus that may be bilateral. Malignant transformation is rare.

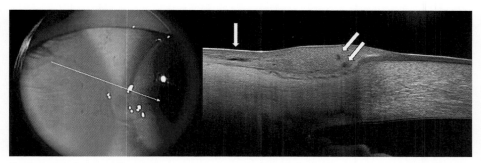

Fig. 16.2 Anterior segment optical coherence tomography (AS-OCT) of a pigmented lesion at the limbus with small cysts *(white arrows)*.

- MM appears as an elevated, unilateral, pigmented lesion with vascularity most commonly located near or crossing the limbus in the temporal quadrant. MM arises from PAM with atypia (most common), from CN (less common), or de novo (less common).
- Ocular melanocytosis appears as grey to brown, flat, pigmented areas. The pigmentation is located on the episclera rather than the conjunctiva, and it therefore will not be freely moveable with the conjunctiva.

WORKING DIAGNOSIS

- Based on the features outlined in the assessment, the lesion may be a CN.
- However, there are features on clinical examination that should raise suspicion for MM.

INVESTIGATION AND TESTING

- Anterior segment optical coherence tomography (AS-OCT) shows the presence of cysts within the pigmented lesion, consistent with CN (Fig. 16.2).
- The pigmented lesion could either be observed over time with routine slit lamp examinations or excised for histopathologic examination.

MANAGEMENT

- Since the gold standard for the diagnosis of CN is excision with histopathologic examination, the pigmented lesion was removed.
- The histopathology report returned confirming the diagnosis of a compound CN.

FOLLOW-UP

- At the 1-month video follow-up post-biopsy, the patient feels well with no pain, irritation, or discomfort in the left eye.

KEY POINTS

- Conjunctival nevi (CN) are benign, variably pigmented lesions of the conjunctiva that are the most common of the conjunctival melanocytic tumors.
- In patients presenting with a pigmented conjunctival lesion, other diagnoses, such as primary acquired melanosis, complexion-associated melanosis, malignant melanoma, and ocular melanocytosis should be considered.

- In cases where cysts are not seen with slit lamp examination, anterior segment optical coherence tomography may be used to identify subclinical cysts that are characteristic for CN.
- The usual management for CN is observation with routine slit lamp examination to monitor for any changes in lesion characteristics, such as size or pigmentation. However, excisional biopsy and histopathology comprise the gold standard for the diagnosis of CN.
- Although CN have a low risk of transformation to malignancy, any change in lesion characteristics should raise suspicion for malignant melanoma, and a biopsy with histopathologic examination should be performed.

CHAPTER 17

Conjunctival Primary Acquired Melanosis Localized

Maya Eiger-Moscovich

Unilateral Pigmented Conjunctival Lesion Involving 2 Clock-Hours in a 58-Year-Old Female

HISTORY OF PRESENT ILLNESS

A 58-year-old White female approached an ophthalmologist 3 months after noticing a pigmented conjunctival lesion in her right eye. The patient was healthy, without ophthalmological history or complaints.

Exam

	OD	OS
Visual acuity	20/25	20/30
IOP (mm Hg)	12	11
Sclera/conjunctiva	Superior conjunctival unifocal pigmented lesion, extending to the limbus and superior cornea, involving 2 clock-hours, from 11:00 to 1:00 Nasal pterygium	White and quiet, nasal pterygium
Cornea	Clear	Clear
AC	Deep and quiet	Deep and quiet
Iris	Brown iris, pupil round	Brown iris, pupil round
Lens	Nuclear sclerosis +1	Nuclear sclerosis +1
Anterior vitreous	Clear	Clear
Retina/optic nerve	Normal optic nerve, posterior and peripheral retina	Normal optic nerve, posterior and peripheral retina

AC, Anterior chamber; *IOP,* intraocular pressure.

QUESTIONS TO ASK

The physician should ask the following questions while assessing the lesion.
- Have the spot changed in size or color?
- Is there any redness or pain?
- Is there a personal history of melanoma?

No financial interest associated with the manuscript. No funding supports.

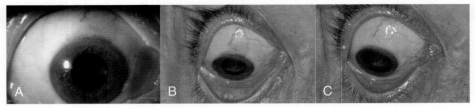

Fig 17.1   (A and B) External photos showing a conjunctival pigmented lesion, extending to the limbus and superior cornea, involving 2 clock-hours, from 11:00 to 1:00. (C) A small stable residual pigmentation at the limbus is observed at follow-up visits.

The patient had not noticed any growth or change in color during the previous 3 months.

The pigmented lesion in the superior conjunctiva was unifocal and freely movable, extending to the limbus and superior cornea, involving 2 clock-hours, from 11:00 to 1:00. The lesion did not contain any cysts, feeding blood vessels, or nodules (Figs. 17.1A–B). There were no other pigmented lesions, including on flipping of the upper eyelid.

ASSESSMENT

- A unilateral unifocal conjunctival pigmented lesion measuring 2 clock-hours and involving the limbus and cornea of a 58-year-old White female.

DIFFERENTIAL DIAGNOSIS

- Primary acquired melanosis, with or without atypia
- Complexion-associated melanosis
- Secondary melanosis
- Conjunctival melanocytic nevus
- Conjunctival melanoma

WORKING DIAGNOSIS

- Right eye localized (under 3 clock-hours) primary acquired melanosis
- Due to White race (there is a tendency to darker skin color in complexion-associated melanosis), lack of accompanying lesions as pterygium (as in secondary melanosis), lack of cysts (as in conjunctival nevus), and lack of feeding blood vessels or nodules (as in conjunctival melanoma)
- The involvement of limbus and cornea raised suspicion for atypia.

INVESTIGATION AND TESTING

- The lesion was documented.

MANAGEMENT

- Excision biopsy was performed. On pathology, primary acquired melanosis with mild atypia, also classified as conjunctival melanocytic intraepithelial neoplasia (C-MIN) grade 2–3, or low-grade conjunctival melanocytic intraepithelial lesion (CMIL) was observed (Fig. 17.2).

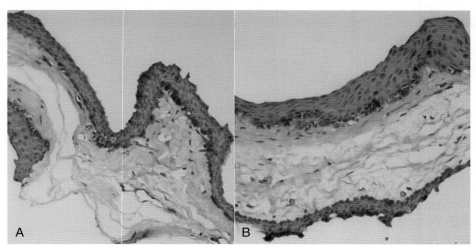

Fig. 17.2 Histopathology photos showing basilar hyperplasia of small normal-appearing melanocytes, with some atypical melanocytes that deviate minimally from normal, diagnosed as primary acquired melanosis with mild atypia, conjunctival melanocytic intraepithelial neoplasia grade 2–3, or low-grade conjunctival melanocytic intraepithelial lesion (stain, hematoxylin-eosin stain, 40x).

FOLLOW-UP

■ After 8 years' follow-up, there was a small stable residual pigmentation at the limbus, with no recurrence or need for further treatment (Fig. 17.1C).

KEY POINTS

■ Primary acquired melanosis should be considered in the evaluation of unilateral or asymmetric conjunctival pigmented lesions.

■ Since level of atypia cannot be determined without pathologic assessment, excisional biopsy should be considered, especially if the lesion is bigger than 3 clock-hours or shows risk factors as feeder vessels, nodules, or involvement of the limbus, cornea, fornix, or tarsal conjunctiva.

■ If atypia is observed on pathologic assessment, the patient should be followed regularly. The frequency of follow-up depends on the level of atypia.

CHAPTER 18

Conjunctival Primary Acquired Melanosis Diffuse

Vijitha S. Vempuluru ■ Carol L. Shields

Diffuse Unilateral Conjunctival Pigmentation in a 76-Year-Old White Female

HISTORY OF PRESENT ILLNESS

A 76-year-old White woman presented with conjunctival pigmentation in her right eye that seemed to increase over 6 months.

Exam

	OD	OS
Visual acuity	20/20	20/20
IOP (mm Hg)	13	11
Sclera/conjunctiva	Extensive pigmentation involving bulbar conjunctiva, superior and inferior forniceal conjunctiva, superior tarsal conjunctiva, and superior eyelid margin (Fig. 18.1)	White and quiet
Cornea	Pigment on 360-degree peripheral 2 mm of cornea	Clear
	Flat pigment 2 mm × 2 mm over central cornea (Fig. 18.1)	
AC	Deep and quiet	Deep and quiet
Iris	Flat freckle at 10:00	Normal color and pattern
Lens	Nuclear sclerosis	Nuclear sclerosis
Anterior vitreous	Clear	Clear
Retina/optic nerve	Normal optic nerve, posterior and peripheral retina	Normal optic nerve, posterior and peripheral retina

AC, Anterior chamber; *IOP,* intraocular pressure.

No financial interest associated with the manuscript.

Support provided in part by the Victoria Cohen Eye Cancer Charitable Trust (Vijitha S. Vempuluru) and the Eye Tumor Research Foundation, Philadelphia, PA, United States (Carol L. Shields). The funders had no role in the design and conduct of the study; in the collection, analysis, and interpretation of the data; and in the preparation, review, or approval of the manuscript.

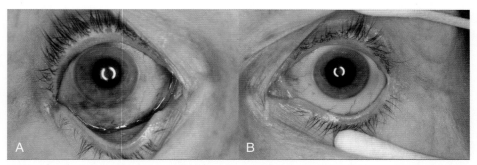

Fig. 18.1 (A) External photograph of the right eye showing diffuse flat conjunctival pigment. (B) Note the complete absence of pigment and normal ocular surface in the left eye.

QUESTIONS TO ASK

- Have you ever noticed any freckles or pigment in either eye?
- Was any procedure or biopsy performed?
- Do you have any personal or family history of skin melanoma?

The patient never had any freckling in either eye. She had not undergone any incisional or excisional biopsy prior to presentation. There is no personal or family history of skin cancer.

ASSESSMENT

- Extensive conjunctival pigment involving bulbar conjunctiva, forniceal conjunctiva, upper tarsal conjunctiva, upper eyelid margin, 360-degree peripheral cornea, and an island of central corneal pigment (Figs. 18.2 A–D).

DIFFERENTIAL DIAGNOSIS

- PAM
- Malignant melanoma
- Complexion-acquired melanosis
- Secondary melanosis

WORKING DIAGNOSIS

- Conjunctival PAM, diffuse – right eye

INVESTIGATION AND TESTING

- Anterior segment optical coherence tomography demonstrated mild epithelial hyperreflectivity of conjunctival epithelium (Fig. 18.2E).

MANAGEMENT

- Patient underwent excision biopsy of thicker pigment at 8:00 limbus, inferior fornix, and superior tarsal conjunctiva with eyelid margin. Cryotherapy was performed to the entire ocular surface with conjunctiva lifted off the sclera to avoid scleral freeze.
- Histopathology revealed PAM with microscopic focus of invasive malignant melanoma.
- In view of residual diffuse corneal and conjunctival pigment, the patient was advised to apply topical mitomycin C eye drops (0.04%) four times a day on a 1 week on and 1 week off regimen, for a total of 2 months.

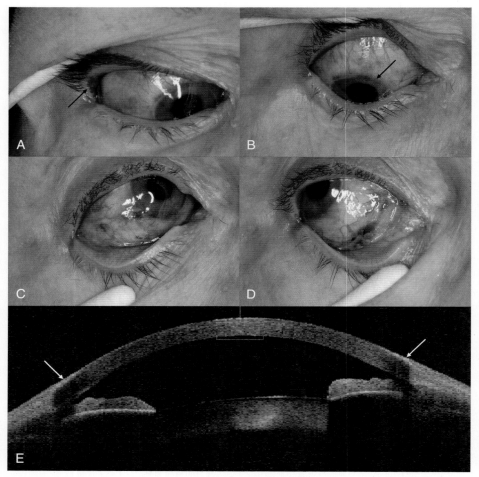

Fig. 18.2 External photographs of the right eye showing diffuse pigment involving 12 clock-hours of bulbar conjunctiva, superior palpebral and tarsal conjunctiva *(arrow)*, eyelid margin (A), peripheral cornea (B, *arrow*), and inferior forniceal conjunctiva (C, D). Anterior segment optical coherence tomography showing mild epithelial hyperreflectivity at limbus and peripheral cornea (E, *arrows*).

- Four months later, there was complete resolution of conjunctival and corneal pigment (Figs. 18.3A–18.3E).

FOLLOW-UP

- At 3-year follow-up, the patient remained tumor free with no recurrence of corneal or conjunctival pigment.

KEY POINTS

- PAM accounts for nearly one-fourth of all pigmented melanocytic lesions involving bulbar, forniceal, or palpebral conjunctiva.
- PAM manifests as unifocal to multifocal, flat epithelial lesions with ill-defined margins, typically unilateral or asymmetric when bilateral.

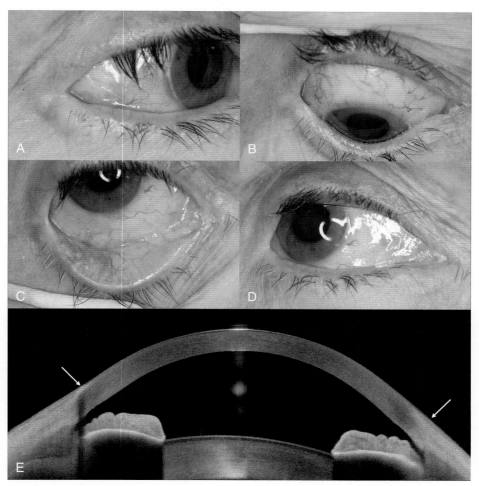

Fig. 18.3 (A–D) External photographs of the right eye showing complete resolution of conjunctival and corneal pigment. (E) Note the restoration of normal epithelial reflectivity on anterior segment optical coherence tomography *(arrows)*.

- Diffuse PAM warrants treatment, and options include surgical excision, cryotherapy, topical chemotherapy with mitomycin-C eye drops or 5-fluorouracil eye drops.
- The first line of treatment in cases with corneal involvement, where amenable, is complete surgical excision by "no-touch" technique and cryotherapy with alcohol keratectomy. Ensuring a dry surgical field is crucial to avoid tumor seeding into healthy ocular surface, and incisional biopsies are contraindicated.
- Mitomycin C (0.01% to 0.04%) is a useful adjunct to surgery and cryotherapy for diffuse PAM. Two to four cycles of medication, typically 1 week on and 1 week off, are recommended to avoid toxicity to the ocular surface.
- Limited literature supports use of interferon alpha-2B for conjunctival PAM.
- PAM without atypia has a low risk of transformation to melanoma, whereas PAM with atypia carries a nearly 50% risk of transformation to malignant melanoma. About three-quarters of conjunctival malignant melanomas arise from preexisting PAM.
- Close monitoring is recommended for early detection of recurrent PAM.

CHAPTER 19

Conjunctival Melanoma—Localized

Joseph DeSimone ■ Philip W. Dockery

Melanotic Conjunctival Lesion in a 65-Year-Old White Male

HISTORY OF PRESENT ILLNESS

A 65-year-old White male with a history of a pituitary adenoma excised 26 years prior presents for evaluation of a pigmented conjunctival lesion. The patient states the lesion has been there since childhood.

Exam

	OD	OS
Visual acuity (cc)	20/25	20/25
IOP (mm Hg)	18	19
Sclera/conjunctiva	15 mm × 15 mm × 3.0 mm melanotic lesion on the temporal interpalpebral bulbar conjunctiva with intrinsic vasculature and feeder vessels, no noted conjunctival melanosis	White and quiet
Cornea	Extension of conjunctival lesion onto cornea from 7:00 to 11:00 with no evident corneal stromal invasion	Clear
AC	Deep and quiet	Deep and quiet
Iris	Flat and round	Flat and round
Lens	Nuclear sclerosis	Nuclear sclerosis
Anterior vitreous	Clear	Clear
Retina/optic nerve	Optic nerve pink and sharp, macula intact, retina flat	Optic nerve pink and sharp, macula intact, retina flat
Lymph nodes	No evidence of preauricular or submandibular lymphadenopathy	No evidence of preauricular or submandibular lymphadenopathy

AC, Anterior chamber; *cc,* with correction; *IOP,* intraocular pressure.

QUESTIONS TO ASK

- Has the patient noticed any change in the size of the lesion?
- Is there any personal or family history of cancer?

No financial interest associated with the manuscript. No funding supports.

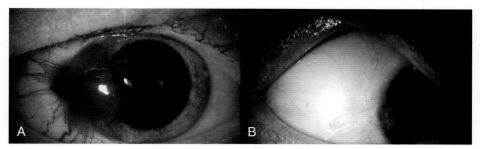

Fig. 19.1 (A) Right eye showing a temporal pigmented conjunctival mass extending over the cornea with intrinsic vasculature and multiple feeder vessels. (B) Slit-lamp image demonstrating white and quiet bulbar conjunctiva with no recurrence 1 year after the initial surgery.

- Does the patient have any other relevant past medical history?

The patient stated that the lesion has been present since childhood, and he does not pay close attention to it, so he is unsure if anything has changed. He presents because of a referral from his primary eye doctor. There is no personal or family history of cancer. Parents deny any other significant past medical history.

ASSESSMENT

- Pigmented conjunctival lesion with corneal involvement, intrinsic vasculature, and feeder vessels, OD (Fig. 19.1A)
- Absence of conjunctival melanosis, OU
- Absence of lymph node enlargement

DIFFERENTIAL DIAGNOSIS

- Conjunctival melanoma
- Conjunctival nevus
- Pigmented conjunctival squamous cell carcinoma

WORKING DIAGNOSIS

- Conjunctival melanoma, OD

INVESTIGATION AND TESTING

- Anterior segment optical coherence tomography (ASO-CT) showed extension onto the cornea with no obvious infiltration of the cornea stroma OD (Fig. 19.2).

MANAGEMENT

- Patient underwent excisional biopsy with 2-mm margins, absolute alcohol corneal epitheliectomy, cryotherapy of the margins and areas of residual pigmentation, conjunctivoplasty, and tissue glue application to promote wound closure.
- Histopathology revealed irregular nests and bands of atypical spindle and epithelioid variably pigmented melanocytes in the substantia propria, associated with prominent increased

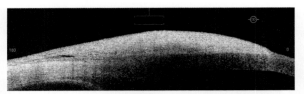

Fig. 19.2 Anterior segment optical coherence tomography (AS-OCT) demonstrating a hyperreflective conjunctival mass extending over the cornea with no apparent invasion of the corneal stroma and no intralesional cysts.

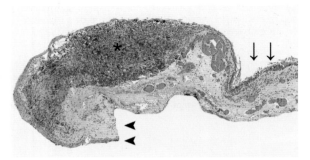

Fig. 19.3 Nodule of invasive melanoma in the substantia propria of the limbal conjunctiva *(asterisk)* adjacent to the melanoma in situ *(arrows)*. Corneal margin *(arrowheads)*.

vascularity, focally severe actinic elastosis, and overlying ulceration, with surrounding intraepithelial proliferation of spindle and epithelioid melanocytes distributing along the basal layer and focally replacing half the epithelial thickness, thus representing invasive malignant melanoma in association with primary acquired melanosis (PAM) with atypia (Fig. 19.3).

FOLLOW-UP

- The patient did not require any further treatment and has remained stable on follow-up for the next year (Fig. 19.1B).

KEY POINTS

- Conjunctival melanoma is a rare melanocytic tumor that arises from nevus, PAM, or de novo.
- While most commonly melanotic and located near the limbus, conjunctival melanoma can be amelanotic, mimicking nonpigmented tumors or metastasis (Fig. 19.4A), or can be hidden in the fornix or palpebral conjunctiva, emphasizing the importance of conjunctival evaluation (Fig. 19.4B).
- Conjunctival melanoma shares similar mutations with cutaneous melanoma (*BRAF, NRAS, NF1, ATRX*), unlike uveal melanoma (most commonly *GNAQ, GNA11*).
- Management of localized conjunctival melanoma requires complete excisional biopsy, with cryotherapy and alcohol epitheliectomy (for corneal involvement). In each quadrant MAP biopsies can be taken to assess for PAM, which in some cases can be amelanotic and difficult to see clinically. Deep scleral invasion can be managed with plaque radiotherapy, and orbital invasion may necessitate exenteration.

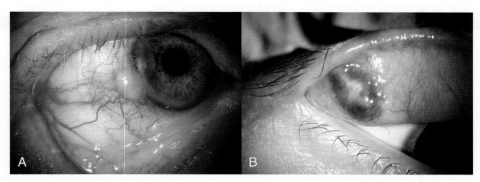

Fig. 19.4 (A) Amelanotic conjunctival melanoma located at the temporal limbus. (B) Melanotic conjunctival melanoma located on the superior tarsus.

- The overall rate of recurrence is 39% at 5 years and 51% at 10 years. The overall rate or metastasis is 16% at 5 years and 22% at 10 years. Rates of metastasis are higher for melanoma located in the fornix or tarsus.

CHAPTER 20

Conjunctival Melanoma Diffuse

Tommy Bui ■ Carol L. Shields ■ Maura Di Nicola

Multiple Conjunctival Lesions in a 48-Year-Old Black Female

HISTORY OF PRESENT ILLNESS

A 48-year-old Black female presents with a fleshy, elevated, pigmented, conjunctival lesion from 10:00 to 11:30 with surrounding dilated vessels and multiple flat pigmented lesions at 3:00, 7:00–9:00, and 12:00. There is also corneal involvement with pigment at 10:00–11:30 (Fig. 20.1). She has noticed these pigmented lesions enlarging in the past few months.

Exam

	OD	OS
Visual acuity	20/25	20/20
IOP (mm Hg)	13	14
Adnexa	Normal eyelids and orbit	Normal eyelids and orbit
Sclera/conjunctiva	Thickened, elevated, pigmented lesion at 10:00–11:30 with surrounding dilated vessels	White and quiet
	Multiple flat pigmented lesions at 3:00, 7:00–9:00, and 12:00	
Cornea	Epithelial invasion with pigment at 10:00–11:30	Clear
AC	Deep and quiet	Deep and quiet
Iris	Unremarkable	Unremarkable
	Brown iris, pupil round, no NVI	Brown iris, pupil round, no NVI
Lens	Clear	Clear
Anterior vitreous	Clear	Clear
Retina/optic nerve	Normal optic nerve, posterior and peripheral retina	Normal optic nerve, posterior and peripheral retina

AC, Anterior chamber; *IOP,* intraocular pressure; *NVI,* neovascularization of the iris.

QUESTIONS TO ASK

- Have the lesions changed in appearance over time? (It is helpful to review old photographs.)
- Is there any personal or family history of cancer?
- Do you have any pain or sensation associated with the lesions?
- Do you have any associated lymphadenopathy?

No financial interest associated with the manuscript. No funding supports.

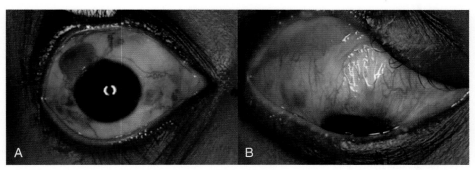

Fig. 20.1 (A) External photograph at baseline showing a fleshy, elevated, pigmented nodule at 10:00–11:30, with surrounding dilated vessels and multiple flat pigmented patches at 3:00, 7:00–9:00, and 12:00. (B) External photograph after surgical excision demonstrates diffuse conjunctival scarring with deep recurrence at 10:00.

The patient has a history of diffuse primary acquired melanosis (PAM). She has noticed the pigmented lesion at 10:00–11:30 enlarging over the past few months. There is no personal or family history of cancer. There is no pain or discomfort associated with the lesions. There is no associated lymphadenopathy.

ASSESSMENT

- Multifocal pigmented conjunctival lesions, OD
- Diffuse conjunctival melanosis, OD

DIFFERENTIAL DIAGNOSIS

- Conjunctival melanoma
- Primary acquired melanosis (PAM)
- Complexion-associated melanosis
- Conjunctival nevi
- Extraocular extension of uveal melanoma
- Distant metastasis of cutaneous melanoma

WORKING DIAGNOSIS

- Diffuse conjunctival melanoma with surrounding primary acquired melanosis

INVESTIGATION AND TESTING

- External/slit lamp photography is helpful in documenting the extent of the conjunctival lesions over time as well as after treatment (Fig. 20.1).
- Anterior segment optical coherence tomography (AS-OCT) demonstrates the subepithelial location of the tumor. Elevated nodules appear hyperreflective with significant posterior shadowing.
- Ultrasound biomicroscopy is utilized to rule out any deep invasion from the conjunctival melanoma to the underlying structures.
- Systemic imaging at baseline and during follow-up is obtained to detect distant metastasis to the lymph nodes and other organs, including the liver and brain.

MANAGEMENT

- Patient underwent alcohol corneal epitheliectomy, surgical removal of the conjunctival lesions, followed by cryotherapy of the margins and placement of an amniotic membrane transplant.
- Histopathology confirmed the presence of diffuse conjunctival melanoma and PAM with severe atypia.

FOLLOW-UP

- After treatment, the patient developed deep recurrence at 10:00, for which she underwent plaque brachytherapy.

KEY POINTS

- Conjunctival melanoma is a rare and potentially life-threatening cancer of the eye that can arise de novo, from PAM or from nevi.
- In patients with PAM with severe atypia, progression to melanoma occurs in up to 50% of cases.
- Management of conjunctival melanoma involves local excision and cryotherapy, based on the extent of disease. Exenteration can be necessary in advanced, invasive cases.
- Diffuse conjunctival melanoma can be particularly challenging to manage, as surgery can be extensive and incomplete resection can increase the risk of recurrence.
- Local tumor recurrence following treatment can be managed with surgery or radiation therapy.
- Patients should be periodically followed to monitor for recurrence and distant metastasis.

CHAPTER 21

Conjunctival Melanoma With Lymph Node Involvement

Hila Goldberg Kremer ■ Bita Esmaeli

New Pigmented Lesion in Bulbar Conjunctiva

HISTORY OF PRESENT ILLNESS

Over the previous 2 months, a previously healthy 27-year-old male noticed a new and growing, elevated, and pigmented lesion in his right lateral bulbar conjunctiva (Fig. 21.1).

QUESTIONS TO ASK

- Do you have have ocular pain or change in vision?
- Do you have any history of surgery or trauma in your right eye?
- Have you noticed any weight loss or any other lesions recently?
- Have you ever had a skin lesion biopsied?
- Have you had unusual UV exposure in the past?
- Is there any history of cancer in your family?

The patient reports a mild burning sensation in the right eye and does not have blurry vision. There are no systemic complaints. He denies previous ocular surgeries, trauma, and skin biopsy. He works as a landscaper, spending about 12 hours outside every day. He denies any family history of cancer.

ASSESSMENT

Exam

	OD	OS
Visual acuity	20/20	20/20
Pupils (dark, light, react, APD)	3, 1, brisk, none	3, 1, brisk, none
IOP (mm Hg)	14	14
External	Palpable preauricular nodule	Normal, no lymphadenopathy
Eyelids	Normal, no pigmentation/lesion on upper lid eversion	Normal, no pigmentation/lesion on upper lid eversion
Sclera/conjunctiva	11-mm nodular pigmented mass in lateral bulbar conjunctiva with extension to lateral limbal cornea	White and quiet
Cornea	Clear	Clear
AC	Deep and quiet	Deep and quiet

No financial interest associated with the manuscript. No funding supports.

Exam—cont'd

	OD	OS
Iris	Round and reactive	Round and reactive
Lens	Clear	Clear
Vitreous	Clear	Clear
Disc	Normal 0.5	Normal 0.5
Retina/macula	Normal	Normal

AC, Anterior chamber; *APD,* afferent pupillary defect; *IOP,* intraocular pressure.

DIFFERENTIAL DIAGNOSIS

- Conjunctival melanoma
- Extraocular extension of uveal melanoma
- Pigmented ocular surface squamous neoplasia (OSSN)
- Conjunctival nevus

WORKING DIAGNOSIS

- Conjunctival melanoma with suspected nodal metastasis

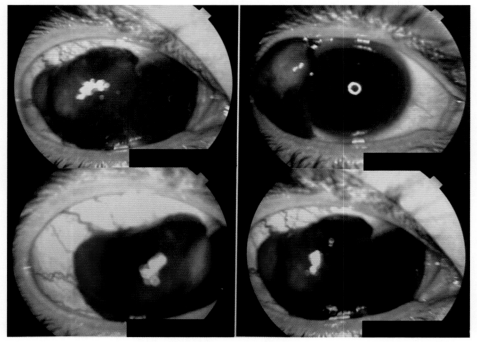

Fig. 21.1   Right eye slit-lamp photos of initial conjunctival lesion.

INVESTIGATION AND TESTING

- Ultrasound (US) head and neck soft tissue: two prominent lymph nodes in superficial right parotid. No other suspicious adenopathy.
- US-guided fine-needle aspiration (FNA) of two suspicious right parotid nodules:
  - Sparse malignant cells consistent with metastatic melanoma
  - Normal lymph node, no abnormal cells identified
- CT chest/abdomen/pelvis: no sign of metastatic disease
- MRI brain: no sign of metastatic disease

MANAGEMENT

- Wide local excision of right conjunctival lesion with cryotherapy to conjunctival margins, alcohol epithelial keratectomy, and conjunctival defect reconstruction with amniotic membrane
- Concurrent right superficial parotidectomy and right neck dissection (levels 1–3)
- Pathology analysis of surgical specimens:
  - Conjunctival melanoma, invasive, mucosal type

Histologic Feature	Result
Tumor thickness	3.9 mm
Mitotic figures	30 mm^2
Ulceration	Present (4 mm)
Predominant cytology	Epithelioid
Regression	Not identified
Vascular/perineural invasion	Not identified
Microscopic satellitosis	Not identified
Associated melanocytic nevus	Not identified
Surgical margins	Peripheral – negative, deep – positive

- Of 36 lymph nodes, 3 were resected and positive for melanoma metastasis (2 superficial parotid and 1 preauricular; all 25 neck nodes were negative)
- Mutation analysis: *BRAF* negative, *NRAS* positive, *KIT* negative
- Adjuvant treatment with pegylated interferon injections for 1 year

FOLLOW-UP

- Postop evaluation at 6 months revealed suspicious subconjunctival nodule in the area of previous melanoma (Fig. 21.2A), worrisome for local recurrence versus scar.
  - Scheduled for excisional biopsy, but due to family reasons it was not done.
  - Completed the excision 3 months later, at which time the lesion had grown (Fig. 21.2B).
  - Pathology analysis of the surgical specimen was positive for melanoma with histologic features similar to the original conjunctival melanoma.
- The patient started suffering from right neck pain 15 months after initial surgery:
  - Neck CT confirmed progressive disease with new right neck nodal metastases (Fig. 21.3).
  - Patient started treatment with ipilimumab/nivolumab immunotherapy (overall for 9 months), with good initial clinical and radiographic response.
- The patient continued his follow-up elsewhere for the next 12 months, without any systemic treatment.
- He returned to our center 12 months later for evaluation of self-palpated right neck mass:
  - Neck CT and US-guided FNA biopsy confirm bilateral cervical positive nodes.

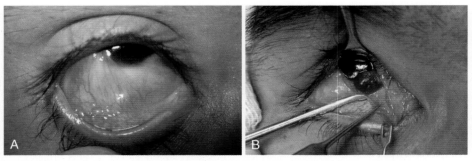

Fig. 21.2 Right eye external photos. (A) Subconjunctival nodule suspicious for recurrent conjunctival melanoma. (B) Three months later: surgical excision of the suspicious subconjunctival nodule.

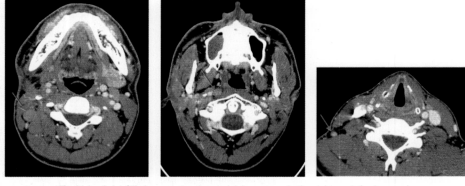

Fig. 21.3 Axial CT shows extensive nodal recurrence in the right neck (*red arrows*).

- Brain MRI and CT of chest/abdomen/pelvis showed no evidence of distant metastases.
- Bilateral neck dissection was completed; pathology results 2/21 right neck and 1/17 left neck lymph nodes were positive for metastatic melanoma.
- The patient started adjuvant treatment with nivolumab.
- On his last follow-up (4 years after initial presentation), the patient was doing well, continuing nivolumab treatment (7 months so far), with no clinical or radiographic signs of local recurrence or metastatic disease.

KEY POINTS

- Conjunctival melanoma is a rare disease with incidence of <1/1,000,000, comprising only 5% of ocular melanomas and <1% of all melanomas.
- The tumor can arise de novo or originate from preexisting nevus or primary acquired melanosis (PAM).
- Conjunctival melanoma differs substantially in histopathology, genetic profile, biological behavior, and management from the more common uveal melanoma and is significantly more similar to the cutaneous melanomas.
- Clinical and histologic features associated with worse prognosis include nonbulbar location, tumor thickness >2 mm, mitotic rate >1/mm^2, presence of ulceration, and epithelioid cell type.
- Conjunctival melanoma is a potentially lethal disease, with a 10-year local recurrence rate as high as 66% and a 10-year mortality rate up to 30%.

- The current mainstay of treatment for local control is wide excision with cryotherapy to margins. Widespread disease may necessitate more extensive surgery, in rare cases even orbital exenteration.
- Alternative or adjuvant local treatment options include topical chemotherapy, brachytherapy, radiotherapy, and, more recently, immunotherapy using immune checkpoint inhibitors.
- Sentinel lymph node biopsy (SLNB) should be considered in cases with a high risk of regional metastasis—that is, tumors thicker than 2 mm or presence of histological ulceration.
- For treatment of metastatic conjunctival melanoma, preliminary clinical data from recent years show promising results for systemic targeted therapy (such as *BRAF* and *MEK* inhibitors) and immunotherapy (such as checkpoint inhibitors anti-CTLA4 and anti-PDL1).

CHAPTER 22

Conjunctival Squamous Cell Carcinoma

Fairooz Puthiyapurayil Manjandavida ■ Kaustubh Mulay

Conjunctival Mass in a 59-Year-Old Male Postsurgery

HISTORY OF PRESENT ILLNESS

A 59-year-old male was referred with a rapidly progressive over 1 month elevated reddish mass in the left eye (OS). He had a previous history of an excision biopsy at the same site 2 years prior. No histopathological confirmation of the diagnosis was available. Postsurgery 1 year he noticed a regrowth of a similar lesion. This rapidly progressed to a nodular mass associated with pain and redness. Systemically he was healthy and immunocompetent.

Exam

	OD	OS
Visual acuity	20/20	20/20
IOP (mm Hg)	12	14

Conjunctiva	Nasal bulbar conjunctival thickening	1. Nodular elevated reddish mass involving the temporal limbus and conjunctiva extending from clock hours 12:00 to 2:30 (Fig. 22.1A–B)
		   - Medial edge conjunctival thickening
		   - Intrinsic vascularity
		   - Multiple large feeder vessels
		   - Specks of keratin at limbus
		   - Rose Bengal staining positive
		   - Immobile
		2. Nasal bulbar conjunctival thickening with scattered pigmentation

Cornea	Clear	Corneal extension from clock-hours 11:30 to 4:00 (Fig. 22.1A)
Sclera	Normal	-Tenderness at clock-hour 2:00 -Mass fixed to sclera
AC	Deep and quiet	Deep and quiet
Iris	Brown, round, regular, and reactive	Brown, round, regular, and reactive
Lens	Nuclear sclerosis: grade 1	Nuclear sclerosis: grade 1
Anterior vitreous	Clear	Clear

No financial interest associated with manuscript. No funding supports.

Exam—cont'd

	OD	OS
Retina/optic nerve	Optic nerve cup disc ratio 0.3, healthy neuroretinal rim, intact fovea, and peripheral retina peripheral retina	Optic nerve cup disc ratio 0.3, healthy neuroretinal rim, intact fovea, and peripheral retina

AC, anterior chamber; *IOP*, intraocular pressure.

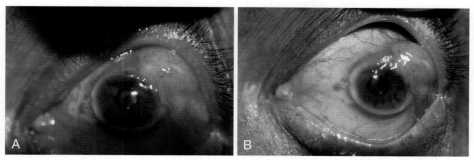

Fig. 22.1 (A) Clinical photograph of the left eye in a 59-year-old male shows a reddish nodular lesion arising from the ocular surface extending from clock hours 12:00 to 2:30 and involving the limbus and conjunctiva. The cornea seems to be involved from clock hours 11.30 to 4.00. It is immobile and fixed to underlying sclera. (B) Multiple feeder vessels are seen with intrinsic vascularity over the surface of the lesion. Specks of keratin are seen in the edge of the mass at clock hour 1:00.

QUESTIONS TO ASK

- Rapidity of the growth of the lesion?
- Associated pain?
- History of previous surgery and histopathology report?
Systemic immunocompromised/immunocompetent status:
- Rapidly progressive conjunctival mass indicates a malignant lesion.
- Ocular surface squamous neoplasia with associated pain clinically indicates invasive squamous cell carcinoma due to scleral involvement.
- Previous surgery indicates a recurrence. It is essential to investigate the previous histopathology report if available. However, in this case the excised lesion was not histopathologically evaluated.
- Aggressive and recurrent pigmented ocular surface squamous neoplasia (OSSN) is common in immunocompromised individuals.

ASSESSMENT

- Conjunctival/limbal nodular elevated reddish mass with intrinsic vascularity, multiple feeder vessels, specks of keratin, and Rose Bengal staining positivity with corneal extension at the previously operated site OS
- Scleral fixity of the mass, OS
- Regional lymph nodes not palpable

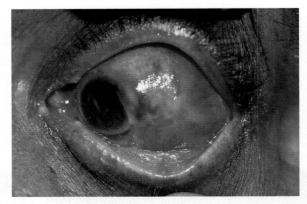

Fig. 22.2 Clinical photograph of the ocular surface postoperative 1 week with amniotic membrane in place after the wide excision.

DIFFERENTIAL DIAGNOSIS

- Conjunctiva, recurrent invasive squamous cell carcinoma OS
- Conjunctiva, recurrent amelanotic melanoma OS
- Conjunctiva, lymphoproliferative lesion OS

WORKING DIAGNOSIS

- Conjunctiva, invasive squamous cell carcinoma, OS

INVESTIGATION AND TESTING

- Anterior segment ocular coherence tomography (AS-OCT) was suggestive of corneal epithelial thickening.
- Ultrasound biomicroscopy (UBM) showed focal scleral invasion.

MANAGEMENT

- Complete surgical excision involved conjunctival wide excision with 4 mm clear margin, alcohol-assisted keratoepitheliectomy with 2 mm margins, lamellar sclerectomy, and double freeze-thaw cryotherapy. Amniotic membrane was used for surface reconstruction (Fig. 22.2).
- Histopathological evaluation showed stratified squamous keratinized epithelium displaying full-thickness dysplasia, and in a large part tumor was seen infiltrating the stroma in the form of cords, sheets, and islands with severe nuclear atypia and high nuclear cytoplasmic ratio. The tumor was seen infiltrating up to the base of the main mass. Margins presented were free of tumor cells. The base tissue presented separately showed atypical cells. Histopathologically it was confirmed as conjunctival invasive squamous cell carcinoma with base invasion (Fig. 22.3).
- Further radiation to the base/surface was delivered with Ruthenium plaque brachytherapy applied over the ocular surface.

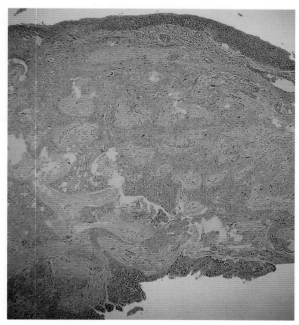

Fig. 22.3 Histopathology PAS section 10x shows thickened conjunctival epithelium with atypical cells invading the stroma arranged as sheets, nests, and cords. The base of the tumor is also involved, suggestive of invasive squamous cell carcinoma of conjunctiva with base positivity.

FOLLOW-UP

- The patient requires strict follow-up every 3 months for the first year, every 6 months for the next 2 years, and yearly thereafter.

KEY POINTS

- Conjunctival OSSN is a neoplastic spectrum including dysplasia, carcinoma in situ, and squamous cell carcinoma.
- Clinical telltale signs aid in differentiating inflammatory and neoplastic mimics from OSSN. Any suspicious lesion of the ocular surface mandates histopathological evaluation postexcision.
- Ultrasound biomicroscopy (UBM) and AS-OCT aid in assessing the anatomical layers involved and the depth of invasion.
- Surgical excision of the tumor with clear margins and base is the treatment of choice in conjunctival squamous cell carcinoma.
- Recurrence is common if the surgical excision does not involve clear margins. Cryotherapy to the margins is an essential step in the surgical management of OSSN to prevent recurrence.
- In the presence of histopathogical confirmation of base involvement, adjuvant focal radiation with plaque brachytherapy is the management protocol for eye salvage to avoid recurrence and intraocular extension.
- Patient should be counseled regarding frequent follow-up to detect early recurrence.

CHAPTER 23

Conjunctival Squamous Cell Carcinoma Recurrent

Hanna Luong ■ Aparna Ramasubramanian

Vascular Elevated Conjunctival Mass in a 68-Year-Old Male

HISTORY OF PRESENT ILLNESS

A 68-year-old male with history of type 2 diabetes and hypertension presents with left eye vascular elevated mass that has been increasing in size for 1 year. He has no prior ocular history or trauma to either eye.

Exam

	OD	OS
Visual acuity	20/50	20/50
IOP (mm Hg)	11	15
Sclera/conjunctiva	White and quiet	Elevated vascular tumor over temporal conjunctiva extending from 12:00 to 7:00 (Fig. 23.1)
Cornea	Clear	Extension of the growth on temporal limbus and cornea
AC	Deep and quiet	Deep and quiet
Iris	Unremarkable	NVI
	Brown iris, pupil round, no NVI	
Lens	Nuclear sclerosis	Clear with visible vascularized retrolental mass
Anterior vitreous	Clear	Clear
Retina/optic nerve	Normal optic nerve, posterior and peripheral retina	Normal optic nerve, posterior and peripheral retina

AC, Anterior chamber; *IOP,* intraocular pressure; *NVI,* neovascularion of the iris.

QUESTIONS TO ASK

- Do you have any pain in the left eye?
- Do you have any bumps anywhere else in your body?
- Do you have any systemic history of immunosuppression?

No financial interest associated with the manuscript. No funding supports.

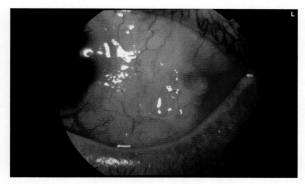

Fig. 23.1 Temporal conjunctiva shows an elevated vascular growth with extension to the limbus and cornea.

The patient has never complained of pain in his OS. He does not have any other bumps in the body, especially no lymph node enlargement by history or on palpation. He has no history of immunosuppression.

ASSESSMENT

- Elevated vascular conjunctival mass, OS

DIFFERENTIAL DIAGNOSIS

- Squamous cell carcinoma
- Amelanotic melanoma
- Lymphoma
- Granuloma

WORKING DIAGNOSIS

- Conjunctival squamous cell carcinoma (cSCC), OS

INVESTIGATION AND TESTING

- B-scan ultrasound of OS showed no obvious scleral involvement
- Optical coherence tomography of OS showed the dense conjunctival lesion with no obvious scleral involvement (Fig. 23.2).

MANAGEMENT

- Patient underwent extensive excision (with partial sclerectomy) with cryotherapy to the edges and amniotic membrane transplant. He also received subconjunctival interferon injection at the time of surgery.
- Histopathology revealed squamous cell carcinoma with negative edges but positive base.
- The patient refused enucleation, and hence external beam radiation was done as globe salvage.

FOLLOW-UP

- The patient had a recurrence (Fig. 23.3) 9 months later that was treated with topical interferon for 1 year.

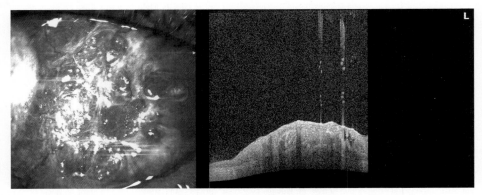

Fig. 23.2 Anterior segment optical coherence tomography (AS-OCT) shows the solid tumor.

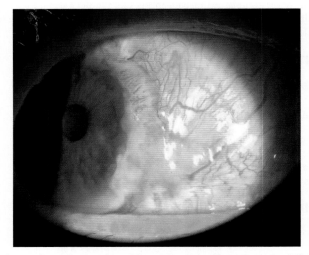

Fig. 23.3 Temporal area shows the scarring of the conjunctiva with a recurrent gelatinous growth on the limbus and cornea.

KEY POINTS

- cSCC is the most common conjunctival malignancy and often manifests at the limbus in the sun-exposed interpalpebral fissure.
- It is associated with male sex, white race, older age, history of prolonged UV light exposure, immunosuppression (i.e., AIDS, xeroderma pigmentosum), and conjunctival infection with HPV 16 and 18.
- Surgical excision with or without cryotherapy is the mainstay of management, but topical therapy such as interferon alpha-2, mitomycin C, and 5-fluorouracil have emerged as primary and adjunctive therapies.
- Plaque radiotherapy and external radiation can comprise an effective alternative to enucleation for residual invasive cSCC and has been associated with a lower risk of local relapse.
- cSCC has a reported 30–41% rate of local recurrence after treatment and 70% and 50% 5- and 10-year overall survival estimates, respectively.

CHAPTER 24

Conjunctiva Lymphoma

Fariba Ghassemi

Fleshy Pinkish Mass on Right Eye Conjunctiva in a 38-Year-Old Male

HISTORY OF PRESENT ILLNESS

A previously healthy 38-year-old Iranian male presented with a pinkish lesion on his right eye that he had first noticed a few months earlier. He reported poor eyesight, slight irritation, a feeling of fullness, and intermittent foreign body sensation in the right eye (Fig. 24.1).

Exam

	OD	OS
Visual acuity	8/10	10/10
IOP (mm Hg)	14	15
Sclera/conjunctiva	A salmon-colored, elevated, gelatinous nasal bulbar conjunctival lesion that expanded to the superior and superotemporal bulbar conjunctiva	White and quiet
Cornea	Clear	Clear
AC	Deep and quiet	Deep and quiet
Iris	Unremarkable	Unremarkable
Lens	Clear	Clear
Anterior vitreous	Clear	Clear
Retina/optic nerve	Normal optic nerve, posterior and peripheral retina	Normal optic nerve, posterior and peripheral retina

AC, Anterior chamber; *IOP,* intraocular pressure.

QUESTIONS TO ASK

- Have you ever had pain in your OD?
- Have you had any recent infection?
- What other medical or surgical conditions have you ever had?
- Is there any history of cancer in your family?
- Does you have any history of using tobacco, alcohol, or illicit drugs?
- Is anything systemic involved?

The patient denied using tobacco, alcohol, or illicit drugs. There was no history of a recent infection or any other medical conditions. The surgical history was negative. The systemic evaluation by the oncologist was negative.

No financial interest associated with the manuscript. No funding supports.

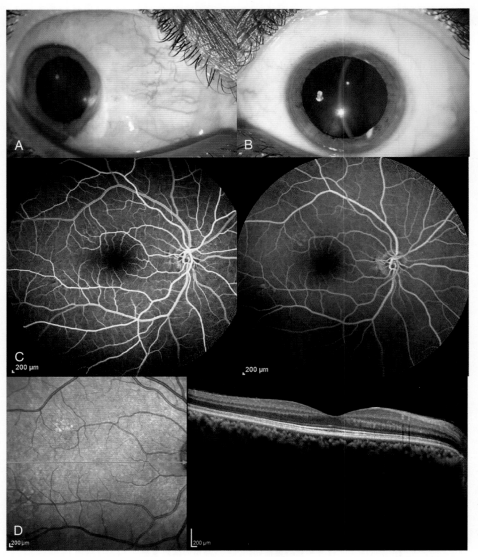

Fig. 24.1 (A) A salmon-patch extensive conjunctival lymphoma with extension of the tumor from nasal side to superior and superotemporal bulbar conjunctiva in the right eye. (B) The left eye was normal. (C) Fluorescein angiography was normal in the early *(left)* and late phase *(right)*. (D) Optical coherence tomography of the fundus was unremarkable.

ASSESSMENT

- A salmon-colored, elevated, gelatinous nasal bulbar conjunctival lesion that expanded to the superior and superotemporal bulbar conjunctiva, OD
- No palpable preauricular, submandibular, or cervical lymph nodes, OD

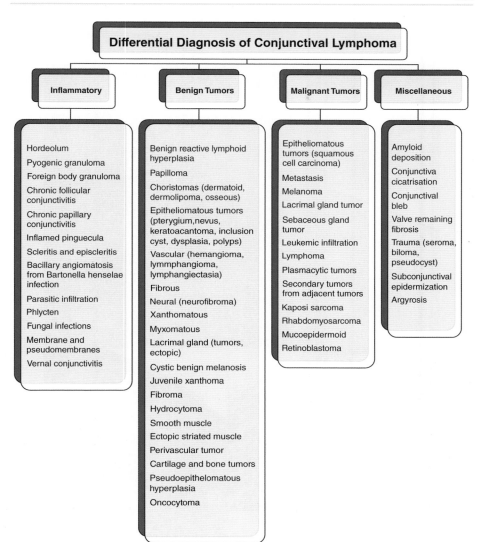

Differential Diagnosis of Conjunctival Lymphoma

Inflammatory	Benign Tumors	Malignant Tumors	Miscellaneous
Hordeolum	Benign reactive lymphoid hyperplasia	Epitheliomatous tumors (squamous cell carcinoma)	Amyloid deposition
Pyogenic granuloma	Papilloma	Metastasis	Conjunctiva cicatrisation
Foreign body granuloma	Choristomas (dermatoid, dermolipoma, osseous)	Melanoma	Conjunctival bleb
Chronic follicular conjunctivitis	Epitheliomatous tumors (pterygium, nevus, keratoacantoma, inclusion cyst, dysplasia, polyps)	Lacrimal gland tumor	Valve remaining fibrosis
Chronic papillary conjunctivitis	Vascular (hemangioma, lymmphangioma, lymphangiectasia)	Sebaceous gland tumor	Trauma (seroma, biloma, pseudocyst)
Inflamed pinguecula	Fibrous	Leukemic infiltration	Subconjunctival epidermization
Scleritis and episcleritis	Neural (neurofibroma)	Lymphoma	Argyrosis
Bacillary angiomatosis from Bartonella henselae infection	Xanthomatous	Plasmacytic tumors	
Parasitic infiltration	Myxomatous	Secondary tumors from adjacent tumors	
Phlycten	Lacrimal gland (tumors, ectopic)	Kaposi sarcoma	
Fungal infections	Cystic benign melanosis	Rhabdomyosarcoma	
Membrane and pseudomembranes	Juvenile xanthoma	Mucoepidermoid	
Vernal conjunctivitis	Fibroma	Retinoblastoma	
	Hydrocytoma		
	Smooth muscle		
	Ectopic striated muscle		
	Perivascular tumor		
	Cartilage and bone tumors		
	Pseudoepithelomatous hyperplasia		
	Oncocytoma		

Fig. 24.2 The differential diagnosis of conjunctival lymphoma.

DIFFERENTIAL DIAGNOSIS

■ The long list of differential diagnoses is addressed in Fig. 24.2.

WORKING DIAGNOSIS

■ Conjunctival lymphoma, OD
■ CL with Ann Arbor Level 1

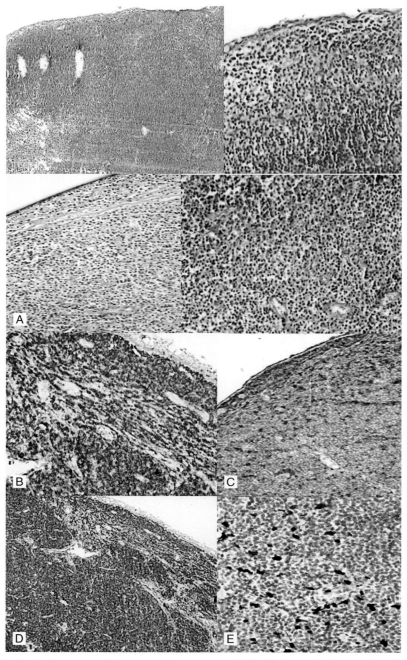

Fig. 24.3 Conjunctival extranodal marginal zone lymphoma (EMZL). (A) Conjunctival tissue with infiltration of small lymphocytes, occasionally exhibits of overt monocytoid cytology, prominent plasmacytic features in the stroma, and epithelium infiltration by lymphoid cells were noted. (B) Immunohistochemistry (IHC) staining shows lymphoid cells' positive reaction for CD20 (B lymphocyte marker). (C) Tumoral lymphoid cells are negative for CD3 (T lymphocyte marker), scattered background T lymphocytes are positive. (D) Diffuse positive reaction for Bcl-2 was observed. (E) A positive nuclear reaction for proliferative marker (Ki-67) showing low-grade lymphoma.

INVESTIGATION AND TESTING

- Incisional biopsy of the mass showed a dense infiltration of small lymphocytes (Fig. 24.3).
- Immunohistochemistry was consistent with extranodal marginal zone lymphoma of the mucosa-associated lymphoid tissue (MALT; Fig. 24.3BE).
- A B-cell monoclonal population with CD20 positivity was found (Fig. 24.3B). CD3 markers were negative, and Bcl-2 and Ki-67 were positive (Fig. 24.3CE).

MANAGEMENT

- The patient received 14 sessions of biweekly subconjunctival rituximab injections for 2 weeks, followed by weekly injection sessions for 4 weeks, four semi-monthly rituximab injections, and two monthly injections into the lesion.
- The lesion regressed mildly but did not disappear.
- The orbit was treated with ultra–low-dose external beam radiation therapy (EBRT) (8 Gy in 4 days) and achieved complete remission after 2 months. The patient has been disease free for the past 2 years.

FOLLOW-UP

- The patient did not require any further treatment and has remained stable on follow-up for 2 years.

Key Points

- CL is a relatively rare, painless, salmon-pink, smooth-surfaced, fleshy patch.
- The conjunctiva is an important site of extranodal lymphoma development, which comprises one-third of all lymphomatous disease.
- CL accounts for roughly one-quarter of all ocular adnexal lymphomas, while being less prevalent than conjunctival squamous neoplasia or melanoma.
- The most prevalent type of CL is extranodal marginal zone lymphoma, which usually has a fair prognosis.
- If not detected or followed properly, the disease may progress systemically.
- Radiation (local or external beam), local or systemic chemotherapy, and immunomodulation are options for treatment.
- The histological subtype of conjunctival lymphoma is an important predictor of outcome.
- MALT lymphomas are thought to be associated with persistent inflammatory or autoimmune diseases.

SECTION 3

Iris and Ciliary Body Tumors

CHAPTER 25

Iris Juvenile Xanthogranuloma

Anthony Mai ■ Marielle P. Young

White Area on the Right Iris in a 2-Month-Old Female

HISTORY OF PRESENT ILLNESS

A previously healthy 2-month-old female presented with a white area on her right inferonasal iris that mom noticed 1 week prior to exam. The initial examination revealed inferonasal right segmental iris heterochromia but otherwise normal anterior and posterior exam. She was initially diagnosed with possible incomplete iris coloboma. However, she returned 6 days later with a new right hyphema.

Exam

	OD	OS
Visual acuity	Fix on light, poor tracking	Fix on light, good tracking
IOP (mm Hg)	20	7
Lids/lashes	Normal	Normal
Sclera/conjunctiva	White and quiet	White and quiet
Cornea	Clear	Clear
AC	4+ heme with layering hyphema	Deep and quiet
Iris	Diffuse inferior bleeding obscuring architecture, lighter iris inferonasally not well visualized	Round and reactive
Lens	Clear	Clear
Anterior vitreous	Difficult view	Clear
Retina/optic nerve	Poor red reflex	Normal red reflex

AC, Anterior chamber; *IOP,* intraocular pressure.

QUESTIONS TO ASK

- Was there any recent trauma?
- Does the patient have any nonocular lesions (i.e., skin)?
- Is there a history of bleeding disorders in either the patient or the family?
- Is there a history of sickle cell anemia in either the patient or the family?
- Does the patient have any other medical conditions?

There was no recent trauma. The patient had two yellow elevated papules on her scalp (Fig. 25.1). There was no history of bleeding disorder or sickle cell anemia in the patient or the family. The patient had no other medical conditions.

No financial interest associated with the manuscript. No funding supports.

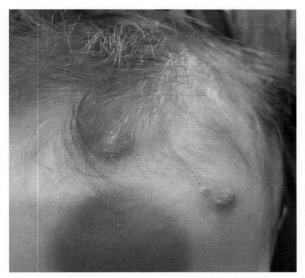

Fig. 25.1 Two yellow elevated papules on the scalp with mild surrounding inflammation.

ASSESSMENT

- Spontaneous hyphema, OD
- Non-pigmented iris lesion, OD
- Scalp papules

DIFFERENTIAL DIAGNOSIS

- Juvenile xanthogranuloma (JXG)
- Amelanotic nevus
- Sarcoidosis
- Leukemia
- Retinoblastoma
- Medulloepithelioma

WORKING DIAGNOSIS

- Spontaneous hyphema secondary to juvenile xanthogranuloma

INVESTIGATION AND TESTING

- Exam under anesthesia showed hyphema (Fig. 25.2)
- Anterior segment B-scan ultrasound: unremarkable
- Ultrasound biomicroscopy: 1 mm × 3 mm right iris lesion with normal ciliary body (Fig. 25.3)

MANAGEMENT

- Hyphema resolved with prednisolone 1% and slow taper and cyclopentolate 1%.
- Recurrent hyphemas occurred 2 and 10 months later, both treated with prednisolone 1% and slow taper.

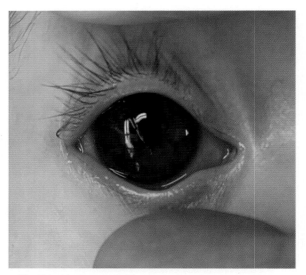

Fig. 25.2 Hyphema with blood at various stages of resolution.

- Intraocular pressure (IOP) was elevated during the third bleed and successfully lowered with Cosopt eye drops.
- Amblyopia OD was managed with patching and glasses.

FOLLOW-UP

- Patient was seen every 3 months over the following year without rebleed.

Key Points

- JXG is the most common non-Langerhans cell histiocytic proliferation that typically affects infants younger than 2 years and regresses by 5 to 6 years of age. Involvement in adults is rare, presenting in the third to fourth decades of life.
- Histologic features include lipid-laden histiocytes, Touton giant cells, and lymphocytes.
- Skin involvement is common and characterized by small, round, tan-orange papules on the face, neck, or torso. The number of skin papules directly correlates with the risk for ocular involvement.

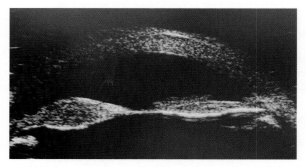

Fig. 25.3 Ultrasound biomicroscopy showing iris thickening suggestive of a lesion (1 mm × 3 mm).

- Eye involvement is rare and characterized by a unilateral localized fleshy brown-yellow iris lesion that may be either nodular or diffusely infiltrative.
- JXG iris lesions typically present with ocular redness and spontaneous hyphema secondary to iris vessel fragility.
- Secondary glaucoma may develop from infiltration of the angle by JXG histiocytes or clogging of the angle from the hyphema.
- JXG responds well to corticosteroids, which often also results in lower intraocular pressure. Depending on the severity, the steroids can be delivered topically, intralesionally, subconjunctivally, or systemically.
- Focal radiation or surgical excision may be considered in cases of vision-threatening sequelae, recurrent hyphema, uncontrolled glaucoma, or lack of response to corticosteroid treatment.
- Patients with iris xanthogranulomas require close observation to track lesion growth, intraocular pressures, and visual behavior.
- Amblyopia can be worsened by prolonged treatment with cycloplegic agents.

CHAPTER 26

Iris Nevus

Sahar Parvizi ■ Guy Simon Negretti

A Pigmented Iris Lesion in a 59-Year-Old Female

HISTORY OF PRESENT ILLNESS

A 59-year-old White female presents with a pigmented right eye iris lesion found on a routine examination by her optometrist. She has right eye amblyopia and had right eye strabismus surgery for an exotropia as a child. She had optic neuritis secondary to relapsing-remitting multiple sclerosis in the same eye.

QUESTIONS TO ASK

- Have you noticed the spot on the iris before, and has there been any change?
- Do you have any history of bleeding in the eye?
- Do you have any personal or family history of cancer?

She had not noticed the spot on the iris before, and there was no history of bleeding in the eye. There was no personal or family history of cancer.

ASSESSMENT

- The patient was assessed at presentation and then again 4 years later.

Exam

	2018	2022
Visual acuity	20/40 OD, 20/17 OS	20/40 OD, 20/20 OS
IOP (mm Hg)	15 OD, 17 OS	18 OD, 19 OS
Iris	A raised pigmented iris lesion (OD) situated close to the pupillary margin at the 2:00 position, measuring 0.8 mm in diameter and 0.5 mm in elevation (Fig. 26.1).	A raised pigmented iris lesion (OD) situated close to the pupillary margin at the 2:00 position, measuring 0.8 mm in diameter and 0.5 mm in elevation (Fig. 26.2).
Angle	No angle seeding	No angle seeding
Posterior segment	Retina flat, macula intact	Retina flat, macula intact

IOP, intraocular pressure.

Figs. 26.1 and 26.2 show the pigmented iris lesion with no ectropion uveae, no feathery margin, no iris seeding, no feeder vessels, and no change over a 4-year period.

No financial interest associated with the manuscript. No funding supports.

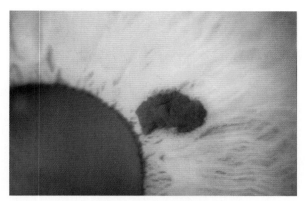

Fig. 26.1 Slit-lamp color photograph of the iris nevus at presentation. A pigmented, raised lesion close to the pupillary margin at the 2:00 position, measuring 0.8 mm in diameter and 0.5 mm in elevation, is noted. There is no associated ectropion uveae, no feathery margin, no pigment seeding, and no feeder vessels.

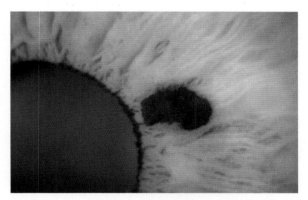

Fig. 26.2 Slit-lamp color photograph of the iris nevus 4 years after presentation. Dimensions remain stable at 0.8 mm in diameter and 0.5 mm in elevation.

DIFFERENTIAL DIAGNOSIS

- Iris nevus
- Iris melanoma
- Iris melanocytoma
- Lisch nodule
- Koeppe and/or Busacca nodule

WORKING DIAGNOSIS

- Iris nevus with no growth over 4 years of follow-up

INVESTIGATION AND TESTING

- Ultrasound biomicroscopy (UBM) at presentation showed a raised lesion at the 2:00 pupil margin, which was 0.5 mm in thickness and had high internal echogenicity (Fig. 26.3). A

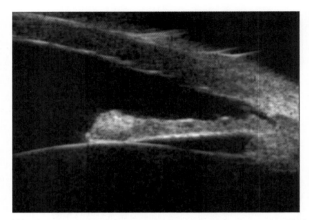

Fig. 26.3 Ultrasound biomicroscopy of the iris nevus at presentation showing a raised lesion at the 2:00 pupil margin, which is 0.5 mm in thickness and has high internal echogenicity.

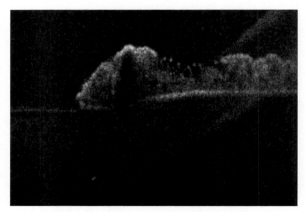

Fig. 26.4 Anterior segment optical coherence tomography (AS-OCT; horizontal section) showing an optically dense iris lesion at the pupillary margin.

horizontal anterior segment optical coherence tomography (AS-OCT) section showed an optically dense iris lesion at the pupillary margin (Fig. 26.4).

MANAGEMENT

- The patient will continue to have regular reviews by an ophthalmologist to ensure that the iris nevus continues to remain stable.

FOLLOW-UP

- The overall risk of growth to melanoma over 15 years is 8%.[1]

KEY POINTS

- The most important risk factors for an iris nevus growing into a melanoma can be identified using the mnemonic ABCDEF:

Age (<40 years)
Blood (hyphema presence)
Clock-hour (inferior)
Diffuse configuration (>3 clock-hours)
Ectropion uveae
Feathery tumor margins

- Additional factors that may be important in predicting growth to melanoma include tumor seeding on the iris or in the anterior chamber angle, feeder vessels, and nodule formation. Serial multimodal imaging is key in monitoring these lesions; basal diameter measurements can be taken on slit lamp; lesions with elevation/depth require UBM and/or AS-OCT. Gonioscopy is used to check for pigment (seeding) in the angle. For indeterminate lesions, biopsy can be an important tool in helping differentiate between iris nevi and melanomas.

Reference

1. Shields CL, Kaliki S, Hutchinson A, Nickerson S, Patel J, Kancherla S, Peshtani A, Nakhoda S, Kocher K, Kolbus E, Jacobs E, Garoon R, Walker B, Rogers B, Shields JA. Iris nevus growth into melanoma: Analysis of 1611 consecutive eyes: The ABCDEF guide. *Ophthalmology.* 2013;120(4):766–772.

CHAPTER 27

Iris Melanoma Nodular

Antonio Yaghy ■ Carol L. Shields

A Growing Pigmented Iris Lesion in a 44-Year-Old Healthy Patient

HISTORY OF PRESENT ILLNESS

A previously healthy 44-year-old white female was referred by her local ophthalmologist for the evaluation of a pigmented iris lesion in the right eye (OD). The lesion has demonstrated an increase in size compared to previous visits. The patient reports excessive tearing, more severe in the right eye, but is otherwise asymptomatic. There is no history of ocular surgery or trauma.

Exam

	OD	OS
Visual acuity	20/20	20/20
IOP (mm Hg)	15	12
Sclera/conjunctiva	1.0 mm × 1.5 mm perilimbal scleral pigmentation along the 2:00 meridian (Fig. 27.1)	White and quiet
Cornea	Clear	Clear
AC	Deep and quiet	Deep and quiet
Iris	4.0 mm × 4.0 mm brown iris lesion from 2:30 to 3:00 meridian (Fig. 27.2)	Within normal limits
Lens	1+ nuclear sclerosis	1+ nuclear sclerosis
Anterior vitreous	Clear	Clear
Retina/optic nerve	Normal optic nerve, posterior retina, and peripheral retina	Normal optic nerve, posterior retina, and peripheral retina

AC, Anterior chamber; *IOP,* intraocular pressure.

QUESTIONS TO ASK

- When did you first notice the pigmented iris lesion, and have you observed any changes in size, shape, or color?
- Have you noticed any other symptoms in the right eye, such as pain, blurriness, or vision loss?

Support provided in part by the Eye Tumor Research Foundation, Philadelphia, Pennsylvania, United States (CLS). The funders had no role in the design and conduct of the study; in the collection, analysis, and interpretation of the data; and in the preparation, review, or approval of the manuscript. Carol L. Shields, MD, has had full access to all the data in the study and takes responsibility for the integrity of the data.

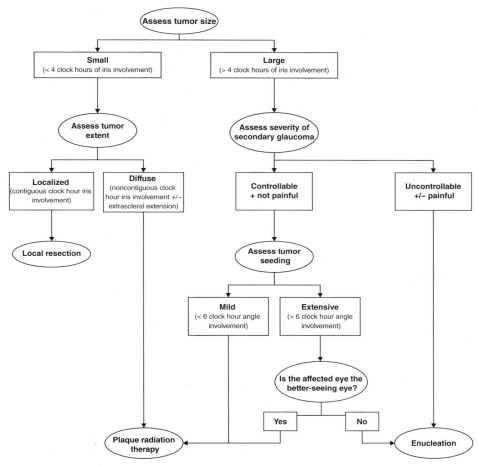

Fig. 27.1 Iris melanoma management algorithm based on tumor size and extent.

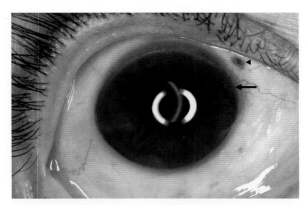

Fig. 27.2 External photograph OD at presentation showing a 4 mm × 4 mm brown iris lesion extending from 2:30 to 3:00 *(black arrow)*. A 1.0 mm × 1.5 mm pigmented perilimbal scleral lesion can also be seen *(black arrow head)*.

- Have you or any member of your family ever been diagnosed with cancer?
- Have you recently noticed any unexplained and involuntary weight loss?

The patient reports that she first noticed the lesion OD 4 years ago and has recently observed that it has increased in size over the past few months. However, she has not noticed any change in shape or color. She denies any other ocular symptoms, has no personal or family history of cancer, and reports no involuntary weight loss.

ASSESSMENT

- Pigmented iris lesion, OD
- Focal scleral pigmentation, OD

DIFFERENTIAL DIAGNOSIS

- Iris melanoma
- Iris nevus
- Iris cyst
- Iris metastasis

WORKING DIAGNOSIS

- Nodular iris melanoma with extrascleral extension

INVESTIGATION AND TESTING

- Ultrasound biomicroscopy OD showed a nodular iris melanoma measuring 3.6 mm in largest basal diameter and 2.6 mm in thickness (Fig. 27.3).
- Anterior segment optical coherence tomography (AS-OCT) OD confirmed the diagnosis and showed an area of scleral thickening at the 2:00 meridian consistent with a focus of extrascleral extension (Fig. 27.4).
- Fine-needle aspiration (FNA) biopsy confirmed the diagnosis of iris melanoma with the perilimbal scleral pigmentation suspicious of extrascleral extension.

MANAGEMENT

- The patient underwent I-125 plaque radiation therapy to the right eye.
- She was referred to a medical oncologist to check liver function twice yearly as well as liver MRI and chest X-ray annually.

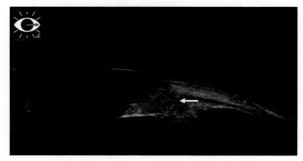

Fig. 27.3 Ultrasound biomicroscopy OD showing an iridociliary melanoma nasally measuring 2.3 mm in thickness and 4 mm in diameter.

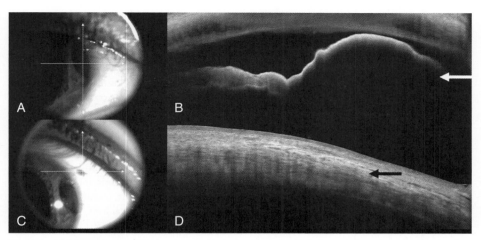

Fig. 27.4 (A) Infrared image OD showing the iris lesion through which the anterior segment optical coherence tomography (AS-OCT) scan was obtained. (B) AS-OCT confirms the presence of the abruptly elevated iridociliary mass *(white arrow)*. (C) Infrared image OD showing the scleral pigment through which a second AS-OCT scan was obtained. (D) The second AS-OCT scan showed mild scleral thickening consistent with extra scleral extension of the tumor *(black arrow)*.

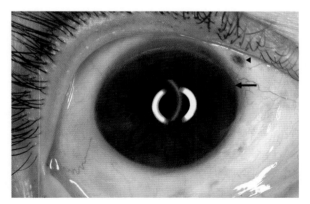

Fig. 27.5 External photograph OD at 7-year follow-up showing a beautifully regressed iris tumor *(black arrow)* and regressed perilimbal scleral pigmentation *(black arrowhead)*.

FOLLOW-UP

- The nodular iris melanoma OD regressed from an original 2.3-mm thickness to a 1.3-mm thickness. The extrascleral extension at the 2:00 meridian regressed beautifully (Fig. 27.5).
- There was no evidence of seeding, angle invasion, or distant metastasis.
- At 3-year follow-up, she developed posterior subcapsular cataract OD at the 2:00 meridian. The cataract was most likely secondary to radiation. To address this, the patient underwent cataract surgery.

KEY POINTS

- Iris melanoma is a rare ocular malignancy and accounts for 4% of all uveal melanomas.
- Risk of metastasis is lower compared to other uveal melanomas, with 7–9% of cases leading to metastatic disease in 10 years.
- Management of iris melanoma depends on clinical features such as tumor size, extent, and location (Fig. 27.1). Uncontrollable or painful secondary glaucoma warrants enucleation.
- The prognosis for iris melanoma varies depending on tumor size and location, as well as other factors such as patient age and overall health. In general, smaller tumors have a better prognosis than larger tumors. The 5-year survival rate for iris melanoma is estimated to be around 90%, but this can vary depending on the individual case.
- It is important to closely monitor patients with iris melanoma after treatment, as there is a risk of tumor recurrence or systemic spread. Yearly ocular examinations and imaging tests should be conducted to detect any signs of recurrence. Additionally, monitoring for metastatic disease may require twice-yearly liver function tests and annual liver MRIs and chest x-rays.

CHAPTER 28

Iris Melanoma Diffuse

Nicholas E. Kalafatis ■ Elliot Cherkas

Iris Neovascularization and Increased Intraocular Pressure in a 64-Year-Old Male

HISTORY OF PRESENT ILLNESS

A 61-year-old male initially presented to his local ophthalmologist with elevated IOP, ectropion uveae, and microcystic edema in the left eye consistent with iridocorneal endothelial syndrome. He underwent successful trabeculectomy shortly after his initial presentation. However, 3 years later the intraocular pressure in his left eye began to rise again, and he was noted to have frank iris neovascularization with thickened amelanotic material on the iris.

Exam

	OD	OS
Visual acuity	20/20	20/20
IOP (mm Hg)	14	20
Sclera/conjunctiva	White and quiet	Extraocular extension at 11:30, scarred bleb superiorly, solid trabeculectomy site at 11:00 potentially filled with tumor, pinguecula at 9:00
Cornea	Clear	Clear
AC	Deep and quiet	Solid mass in angle at 3:00, neovascularization of the angle
Iris	Unremarkable Blue iris, pupil round, no NVI	NVI, 360-degree ectropion iridis, diffuse iris melanoma, peripheral iridotomy at 11:30
Lens	1+ NS	1+ NS
Anterior vitreous	Clear	Clear
Retina/optic Nerve	Normal optic nerve, posterior and peripheral retina	1+ disc pallor, shallow cup, hazy view

AC, Anterior chamber; IOP, intraocular pressure; NS, nuclear sclerosis; NVI, neovascularization of the iris.

QUESTIONS TO ASK

- When did you first notice a change in your eye?
- Do you have any past medical history of skin cancer or melanoma?
- Is there any history of cancer in your family?

No financial interest associated with the manuscript. No funding supports.

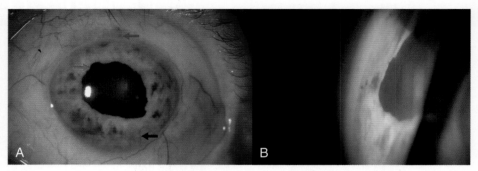

Fig. 28.1 (A) Slit-lamp photograph of the left eye demonstrating diffuse iris melanoma with ectropion uveae *(red arrow)*, iris neovascularization *(black arrow)*, and extraocular extension *(blue arrow)*. (B) Gonioscopy of the left eye showing tumor seeding to the angle.

The patient first noticed brown spots in his left eye 25 years ago but was not diagnosed with glaucoma until 3 years ago. He has no prior history of skin cancer or melanoma. His family history is significant for prostate cancer in his father and brother.

ASSESSMENT

- Diffuse iris pigmentation, OS
- Iris neovascularization, OS
- Ectropion uveae, OS
- Scleral extraocular extension, OS

DIFFERENTIAL DIAGNOSIS

- Iris melanoma diffuse
- Primary iris cyst
- Iris nevus
- Iris metastasis
- Iridocorneal endothelial syndrome

WORKING DIAGNOSIS

- Diffuse iris melanoma with neovascularization of the iris (NVI), angle closure glaucoma, and scleral extraocular extension, OS

INVESTIGATION AND TESTING

- Slit-lamp photographs were taken (Fig. 28.1A) depicting the left eye with diffuse iris melanoma.
- Gonioscopy was performed (Fig. 28.1B), which revealed a mass in the angle and tumor seeding 360 degrees.
- Ultrasound biomicroscopy demonstrating a solid mass in the angle (*white arrow*) consistent with iris melanoma (Fig. 28.2).

MANAGEMENT

- Patient underwent enucleation of the left eye followed by CyberKnife radiotherapy of the orbit.

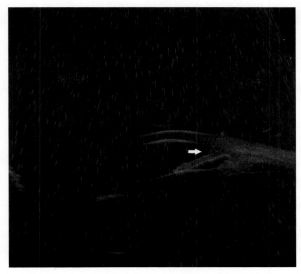

Fig. 28.2 Ultrasound biomicroscopy of the left eye revealing a solid mass in the angle *(white arrow)*.

- Histopathology revealed malignant melanoma of the iris; diffuse, mixed cell type with obstruction of anterior chamber angle; infiltration of trabecular meshwork; and infiltration of anterior emissarial canals and anterior face of ciliary body.
- Orbital biopsies were negative for tumor infiltration of the orbit.

FOLLOW-UP

- The patient returned for his 1-year follow-up and was screened with MRI, which showed no brain metastasis.
- He returned 5 years later after an MRI showed a lesion on the frontal lobe.
- The following year, he developed brain metastases and, despite whole brain radiation, progressed to have metastasis of the liver, kidney, and peritoneum.

KEY POINTS

- Asymmetric iris pigmentation should raise suspicion enough to perform a more thorough evaluation.
- Iris nevus has a 5% rate of transformation into melanoma.
- Patients with lighter-colored irises have increased risk of developing iris melanoma.
- Secondary glaucoma is present in one-third of cases, usually as a result of angle invasion, neovascularization, or hyphema.
- Fine-needle aspiration (FNA) biopsy can be useful to confirm the diagnosis, and genetic testing can be useful to determine prognosis and metastatic potential.
- The most common genetic mutations seen in iris melanoma are *BRAF, GNAQ/GNA11*, and *EIF1AX*.
- Management depends on the size and extent of seeding, with smaller tumors able to be locally resected and larger tumors often requiring plaque radiotherapy or enucleation.

CHAPTER 29

Iris Pigment Epithelial Cyst

Mona Camacci ■ Vikas Khetan

Asymptomatic Iris Lesion With Progression in Size

HISTORY OF PRESENT ILLNESS

A 73-year-old female presents for cataract evaluation. She has a known history of pigment dispersion syndrome, for which she is being monitored. At the time of cataract evaluation, a lesion adjacent and posterior to the inferior iris was noticed. Patient underwent cataract extraction of both eyes without any complications. During optometry 5 years later, the inferior iris mass was enlarged. Patient is asymptomatic.

Exam

	OD	OS
Visual acuity	20/20	20/20
IOP (mm Hg)	14	14
Sclera/conjunctiva	White and quiet	White and quiet
Cornea	Krukenberg spindle on posterior cornea, anterior basement membrane dystrophy	Krukenberg spindle on posterior cornea, anterior basement membrane dystrophy
AC	Deep and quiet	Deep and quiet
Iris	Posterior iris cyst inferiorly, larger compared to previous examination	Small posterior iris cyst temporally that appears regressed
Lens	Posterior chamber intraocular lens in good position	Posterior chamber intraocular lens in good position
Anterior vitreous	Clear	Clear
Retina/optic nerve	Normal optic nerve with cup-to-disc ratio of 0.5, posterior and peripheral retina normal	Normal optic nerve with cup-to-disc ratio of 0.5, posterior and peripheral retina normal

AC, Anterior chamber; *IOP,* intraocular pressure.

QUESTIONS TO ASK

- Do you have any history of ocular trauma?
- Do you have any history of ocular surgery?
- Do you have any history of use of ocular miotics (phospholine iodide) or prostaglandins?

The patient denies any history of ocular trauma. She has never used any ocular eye drops other than artificial tears. She reports bilateral cataract extraction with intraocular lens placement 5 years ago without any complications.

No financial interest associated with the manuscript. No funding supports.

ASSESSMENT

- Cystic lesion posterior to the iris suggestive of primary iris pigment epithelial cyst

DIFFERENTIAL DIAGNOSIS

- Primary iris pigment epithelial or stromal cyst
- Iris nevus
- Iris melanocytosis
- Iris melanocytoma
- Lisch nodule
- Iris or ciliary body melanoma
- Iris pigment epithelium adenoma
- Medulloepithelioma

WORKING DIAGNOSIS

- Primary iris pigment epithelial or stromal cyst

INVESTIGATION AND TESTING

- Dilated depressed fundus examination
- Serial slit-lamp photographs (Fig. 29.1)

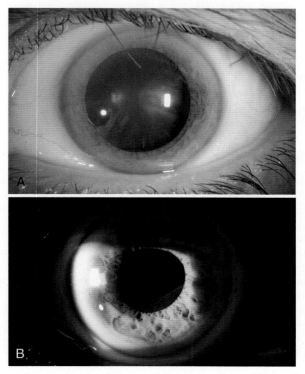

Fig. 29.1 (A) Slit-lamp photograph of the right eye at initial presentation and (B) at subsequent follow-ups 2 years later showing an inferior nasal mass extending from the iris and increasing in size over time.

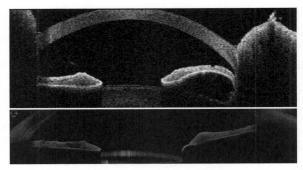

Fig. 29.2 Anterior segment optical coherence tomography at (A) initial presentation and (B) subsequent follow-up presentation showing intranasal cystic lesion posterior to the iris causing bowing forward of the iris.

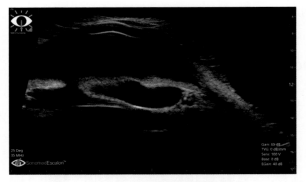

Fig. 29.3 Ultrasound biomicroscopy of the right eye at subsequent follow-up appointments showing enlargement of the cystic lesion.

- Anterior segment optical coherence tomography (AS-OCT) (Fig. 29.2)
- Ultrasound biomicroscopy (UBM) (Fig. 29.3)

MANAGEMENT

- Iris cysts that are asymptomatic and not causing any secondary complications can be followed regularly with serial examinations.
- Iris cysts that are causing secondary complications (angle-closure glaucoma, plateau iris syndrome, glaucoma secondary to pigment dispersion syndrome, corneal edema, lens subluxation, iritis) necessitate intervention.
- Laser treatment with argon laser photocoagulation and Nd:Yag can be used to disturb the production of cystic fluid or to perforate and release the cyst.
- Cyst aspiration with injection of sclerosing agent, such as trichloroacetic acid, 5-fluorouracil, and mitomycin C, can be performed.
- A more aggressive surgical approach would involve excision of the iris cyst with possible use of cryotherapy.

FOLLOW-UP

- Patient was followed up every 3 to 4 months and was stable.

KEY POINTS

- Primary iris cysts can be monitored without intervention.
- If secondary complication such as amblyopia in children, angle-closure glaucoma, plateau iris syndrome, progression of glaucoma secondary to pigment dispersion syndrome, lens subluxation, or iritis occur, then laser or surgical intervention may be necessary.

Ciliary Body Medulloepithelioma

Alex H. Brown ▪ Aparna Ramasubramanian

Leukocoria and Decreased Visual Acuity in a 3-Year-Old Female

HISTORY OF PRESENT ILLNESS

A previously healthy 3-year-old female presents with left eye leukocoria. Her mother commented that the child had seemed unable to notice or track objects on her left side over the previous few weeks. The family also noticed a white glow in the pupil. The child has no prior ocular history or trauma to either eye.

Exam

	OD	OS
Visual acuity	Fix and follow	Fixes briefly
IOP (mm Hg)	11	25
Sclera/conjunctiva	White and quiet	White and quiet
Cornea	Clear	Clear
AC	Deep and quiet	Deep and quiet
Iris	Unremarkable	NVI
	Brown iris, pupil round, no NVI	
Lens	Clear	Clear with visible vascularized retrolental mass
Anterior vitreous	Clear	Vascularized yellow mass with vitreous hemorrhage (Fig. 30.1)
Retina/optic nerve	Normal optic nerve, posterior and peripheral retina	No view of optic nerve
		Vascularized mass covering entire vitreous cavity

AC, anterior chamber; *IOP,* intraocular pressure; *NVI,* neovascularization of the iris.

QUESTIONS TO ASK

- Has your daughter ever had redness or pain in her left eye?
- Is there any history of cancer in your family?
- Does your child have any other relevant past medical history?

The patient has never complained of pain in her left eye. No signs of redness in both eyes. There is no history of cancer in the family. Parents deny any other significant past medical history.

No financial interest associated with the manuscript. No funding supports.

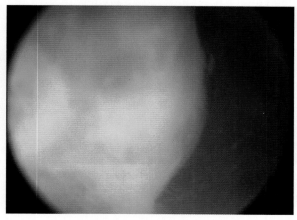

Fig. 30.1 Left eye showing a vascularized yellow mass filling the vitreous cavity with vitreous hemorrhage.

ASSESSMENT

- Vascularized retrolental mass, OS
- Neovascularization of the iris (NVI), OS

DIFFERENTIAL DIAGNOSIS

- Medulloepithelioma
- Retinoblastoma
- Coats disease
- Persistent hyperplastic primary vitreous (PHPV)

WORKING DIAGNOSIS

- Ciliary body medulloepithelioma with NVI, OS

INVESTIGATION AND TESTING

- B-scan ultrasound of OS showed a large peripheral mass arising from the ciliary body that covered almost the entire vitreous cavity (Fig. 30.2A).
- Fluorescein angiogram of OS showed NVI and a large vascularized retrolental mass (Fig. 30.2B).

MANAGEMENT

- Patient underwent enucleation of OS.
- Histopathology revealed a large mass arising from the ciliary body that displayed basophilic cells forming ribbons and tubes with interspersed largely dilated vessels and cysts (Fig. 30.3A–B).

FOLLOW-UP

- The patient did not require any further treatment and has remained stable on follow-up for 4 years.

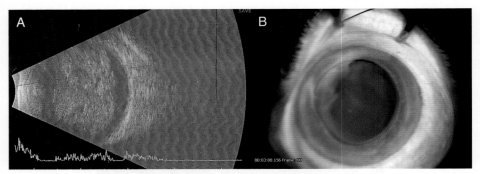

Fig. 30.2 (A) Ultrasound showing a large mass arising from the ciliary body and covering almost the entire vitreous cavity. (B) Fluorescein angiography showing neovascularization of the iris and a vascularized retro-lental mass.

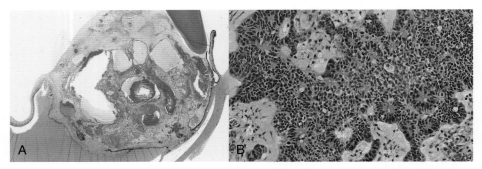

Fig. 30.3 (A) Large mass arising from the ciliary body that has basophilic cells forming ribbons and tubes with interspersed largely dilated vessels and cysts. (B) Round, small, and deeply basophilic tumor cells with some retinoblastoma differentiation. Multiple mitotic figures were present, diagnostic of a malignant nonteratoid medulloepithelioma.

KEY POINTS

- Intraocular medulloepitheliomas are rare, slow-growing, sporadic tumors of the nonpigmented ciliary epithelium.
- Medulloepithelioma has a known association with pleuropulmonary blastoma family tumor and dysplasia syndrome (PPB-FTDS) in approximately 5% of cases.
- Management of advanced ciliary body medulloepithelioma requires enucleation. Local resection of smaller tumors occupying less than 3 to 4 clock-hours is possible, but high rates of recurrence have been reported. Plaque brachytherapy has been successfully used in small to medium-size tumors.
- The prognosis for these patients is generally good if the tumor stays confined to the globe.

CHAPTER 31

Ciliary Body Adenoma (Epithelioma)

Christina Stathopoulos ▓ Alexandre Moulin ▓ Ann Schalenbourg ▓ Carol L. Shields

Retrolental Mass in a 41-Year-Old Female

PRESENTING ILLNESS

Asymptomatic sectorial cataract with retrolental mass discovered after a minor eye trauma.

HISTORY OF PRESENT ILLNESS

A previously healthy 41-year-old female was diagnosed with a sectorial cataract and an intraocular mass while being examined for a minor trauma (son's finger poked her in the left eye).

Exam

	OD	OS
Visual acuity	10/10	10/10
IOP (mm Hg)	15	15
Sclera/conjunctiva	White and quiet	White and quiet
Cornea	Clear	Clear
AC	Deep and quiet	Deep and quiet
Iris	Brown iris, pupil round, no NVI	Brown iris, pupil round, no NVI
Lens	Clear	Sectorial inferonasal cataract
Anterior vitreous	Clear	Retrolental discretely vascularized whitish mass at the level of the ciliary body, facing the lens opacities (Fig. 31.1)
Retina/optic nerve	Normal optic nerve, posterior and peripheral retina	Normal optic nerve, posterior and peripheral retina

AC, Anterior chamber; *IOP,* intraocular pressure; *NVI,* neovascularization of the iris.

QUESTIONS TO ASK

- Do you have any previous history of eye injury or any other past eye examinations?
- Do you experience redness or pain in your left eye?
- Is there any history of cancer in your family?

There has been no previous eye examination that the patient remembers. She reports no symptoms of redness, pain, or any other complaint concerning her OS. There is no history of cancer in the family.

No financial interest associated with the manuscript. No funding supports.

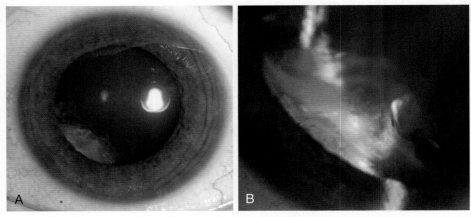

Fig. 31.1   (A) Retrolental vascularized whitish mass with (B) sectorial inferonasal cataract.

ASSESSMENT

- Fine vascularized nonpigmented retrolental mass, OS
- Sectorial cataract

DIFFERENTIAL DIAGNOSIS

- Nonpigmented ciliary body adenoma/adenocarcinoma
- Ciliary body melanoma
- Leiomyoma
- Schwannoma
- Metastasis

WORKING DIAGNOSIS

- Nonpigmented ciliary body adenoma or adenocarcinoma, OS

INVESTIGATION AND TESTING

- No anterior segment invasion was revealed in 360-degree gonioscopy.
- Ultrasound biomicroscopy (UBM) (20 MHz) showed a 4.6-mm-thick mass arising from the surface of the ciliary body (Fig. 31.2A).

MANAGEMENT

- Diagnosis of a ciliary body adenoma was confirmed following a biopsy under lamellar scleral flap, disclosing cords of cuboidal cells surrounded by a network of periodic acid Schiff (PAS)-positive basal membranelike material (Fig. 31.3). Neither significant atypia nor necrosis could be identified.
- Taking into account the size of the tumor, the perfect vision, and the fact that a current adenocarcinoma could not be excluded with an incisional biopsy, nor could the possibility of a malignant transformation in the future, the decision to treat this tumor conservatively was made.
- This tumor was treated with proton beam irradiation (60 Gy), and it regressed to a 1-mm-thick lesion, only visible on UBM (Fig. 31.2B).

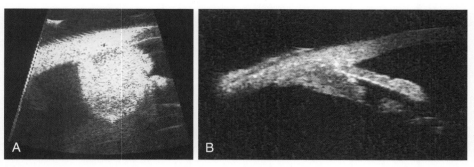

Fig. 31.2 (A) Ultrasound biomicroscopy showed a homogenous mass arising from the ciliary body. (B) Ultrasound biomicroscopy following proton beam irradiation showed a regressed lesion.

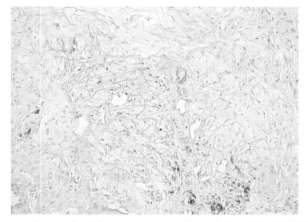

Fig. 31.3 Biopsy revealed cords of cuboidal cells surrounded by periodic acid Schiff (PAS)-positive material.

- The patient developed a cataract 1 year later, which was managed with phacoemulsification and intraocular lens implantation.

FOLLOW-UP

- No regrowth of the lesion was observed, and best-corrected visual acuity remained at 1.0 with no further treatments over a 14-year follow-up.

KEY POINTS

- Ciliary body adenoma is a rare tumor that can be pigmented or nonpigmented.
- Differential diagnosis from adenocarcinoma can be challenging when only based on the clinical signs and/or results of an incisional biopsy.
- In eyes with useful vision, conservative management includes observation for small asymptomatic lesions, surgical resection (sectorial iridocyclectomy), or radiation therapy.
- Large tumors with no visual potential, concomitant glaucoma, or other complications may require enucleation. Exteriorization is anecdotal.
- Regular follow-up is recommended in eyes treated conservatively.
- Survival is excellent in cases with lesions confined to the globe.

SECTION 4

Uveal Pigmented Tumors

SECTION OUTLINE

CHAPTER 32

Choroid Nevus

Kushal Umeshbhai Agrawal ■ Carol L. Shields

Pigmented Choroidal Lesion in the Right Eye (OD) of a 67-Year-Old Male

HISTORY OF PRESENT ILLNESS

A 67-year-old White male was seen for follow-up examination of the pigmented choroidal lesion in the right eye (OD). He was diagnosed to have a choroidal nevus in 1978 and was not having any visual complaints. Left eye (OS) was enucleated due to chronic retinal detachment associated with neovascular glaucoma.

Exam

	OD	OS
Visual acuity	20/20	NA
IOP (mm Hg)	12	NA
Sclera/conjunctiva	White and quiet	Quiet socket
Cornea	Clear	NA
AC	Deep and quiet	NA
Iris	Unremarkable	NA
	Blue iris, pupil round, no NVI	
Lens	Clear	NA
Anterior vitreous	Clear	NA
Retina/optic nerve	Normal optic nerve and macula	NA
	Pigmented choroidal lesion around 7 mm in vertical and 4 mm in horizontal dimensions with overlying drusen	

AC, anterior chamber; *IOP,* intraocular pressure; *NA,* not applicable.

QUESTIONS TO ASK

- Do you have any symptoms?
- Do you have any personal history of cancer?
- Do you have any history of cancer in your family?

The patient does not have any symptoms and does not have personal or family history of cancer.

No financial interest associated with the manuscript. No funding supports.

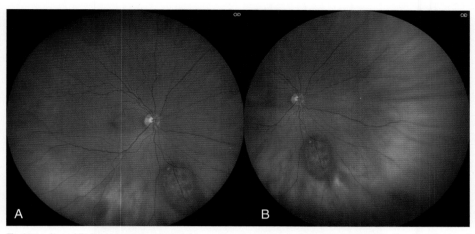

Fig. 32.1 (A and B) Fundus photo of the right eye showing pigmented choroidal lesion with 7-mm vertical and 4-mm horizontal dimensions with overlying drusen.

ASSESSMENT

- Pigmented elevated choroidal lesion inferiorly OD
- Drusen overlying lesion and no clinically visible SRF OD

DIFFERENTIAL DIAGNOSIS

- Choroidal nevus
- Choroidal melanoma
- Choroidal metastasis
- Retinal pigment epithelium (RPE) adenoma

WORKING DIAGNOSIS

- Choroidal nevus OD

INVESTIGATION AND TESTING

- Fundus photo of OD showed pigmented choroidal lesion inferiorly that measured 7 mm in horizontal and 4 mm in vertical dimensions with overlying drusen (Fig. 32.1).
- Autofluorescence of the choroidal lesion showed hypoautofluorescence and absence of orange pigments (Fig. 32.2).
- Optical coherence tomography (OCT) scan of OD showed intact macula and elevation of the retina–choroid complex in the area of choroidal nevus with no SRF (Fig. 32.3).
- Ultrasound scan of OD showed echodense choroidal lesion that was 1.95 mm in thickness with attached overlying retina (Fig. 32.4).

MANAGEMENT

- Patient was asked to follow up every 6 months.

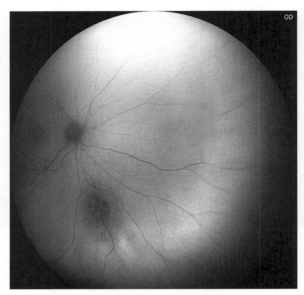

Fig. 32.2 Autofluorescence of the right eye through the lesion, showing relative hypoautofluorescence with absent orange pigments.

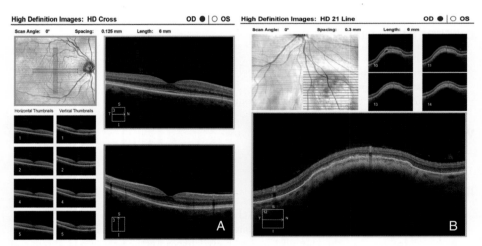

Fig. 32.3 (A) Optical coherence tomography (OCT) scan of the right eye showing intact macula and absence of any subretinal fluid (SRF). (B) OCT scan through the lesion showing elevation of the retina–choroid complex due to choroidal lesion with no SRF.

FOLLOW-UP

- On every follow-up, the following parameters will be assessed: tumor thickness and size, presence or absence of SRF, symptoms, orange pigments, and ultrasound characteristics of the lesion. Patient has been followed up for 34 years to now with no major changes in the lesion.

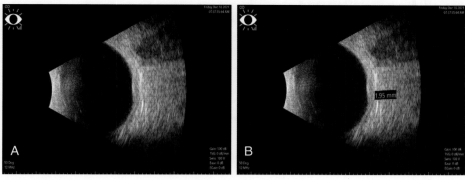

Fig. 32.4   (A) Right eye ultrasound B-scan showing relatively echodense choroidal lesion, inferior to the optic nerve and (B) 1.95 mm thick.

KEY POINTS

- Choroidal nevus is a benign choroidal lesion that can be observed without any further treatment in the majority of cases.
- Choroidal nevus should be differentiated from choroidal melanoma; the latter is a malignant tumor with high metastatic potential and could be life threatening.
- Differentiation of choroidal nevus with choroidal melanoma can be done based on tumor characteristics, using the mnemonic TFSOMDIM:

T = Thickness of the lesion greater than 2 mm

F = Fluid present around lesion

S = Symptoms (patient can have symptoms such as flashes, floaters, diminution of vision, etc.)

O = Orange pigments (presence of orange pigments indicates active disease)

M = Melanoma hollowness on ultrasound scan (choroidal melanoma is acoustically hollow on ultrasound scan, whereas choroidal nevus is acoustically dense)

DIM = Diameter of the lesion more than 5 mm

Among these risk factors, the most important three are thickness, fluid, and orange pigments. Presence of more risk factors points toward the higher risk of conversion of choroidal nevus to choroidal melanoma. Our patient had only one positive risk factor: diameter more than 5 mm.

CHAPTER 33

CHOROID NEVUS WITH SUBRETINAL FLUID

Zeynep Bas

Decreased Visual Acuity and Floaters in a 61-Year-Old Female

HISTORY OF PRESENT ILLNESS

A 61-year-old White female presented with a 2-week history of blurred vision in the left eye (OS). She reported no prior ocular problems, and her medical history was negative.

Exam

	OD	OS
Visual acuity	20/20	20/100
IOP (mm Hg)	14	18
Sclera/conjunctiva	White and quiet	White and quiet
Cornea	Clear	Clear
AC	Deep and quiet	Deep and quiet
Iris	Unremarkable	Unremarkable
	Brown iris, pupil round, no NVI	Brown iris, pupil round, no NVI
Lens	Nuclear sclerosis	Nuclear sclerosis
Anterior vitreous	Clear	Clear
Retina/optic nerve	Normal optic nerve, posterior and peripheral retina	Normal optic nerve, choroidal mass in the macular region (Fig. 33.1)

AC, Anterior chamber; *IOP,* intraocular pressure; *NVI,* neovascularization of the iris.

QUESTIONS TO ASK

- Did the patient have a past retinal examination and/or fundus pictures?
- Does the patient have any other relevant past medical history?

The patient stated that she has not been dilated before. The patient denied any other significant past medical history.

No financial interest associated with manuscript. No funding supports.

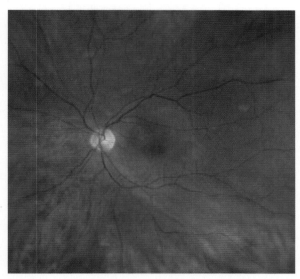

Fig. 33.1 Small choroidal nevus centered in the foveal region. Note the subtle ring of subretinal fluid affecting macula temporally.

ASSESSMENT

- Choroidal mass, OS
- Subretinal fluid, OS
- Leakage in the macular area on fluorescein angiography, OS

DIFFERENTIAL DIAGNOSIS

- Choroidal nevus with subretinal fluid
- Choroidal melanoma
- Choroidal metastasis

WORKING DIAGNOSIS

- Choroidal nevus with subretinal fluid

INVESTIGATION AND TESTING

- B-scan ultrasound of OS showed a flat mass with medium acoustic solidity measuring 2.2 mm in thickness (Fig. 33.2).
- OCT showed choroidal nevus with overlying SRF and retracted photoreceptors (Fig. 33.3).
- Fluorescein angiography in venous phase demonstrated multiple foci of hyperfluorescence representing leakage points (Fig. 33.4).

MANAGEMENT

- Management with three injections of anti-VEGF (generic name: bevacizumab, brand name: Avastin) was provided monthly.

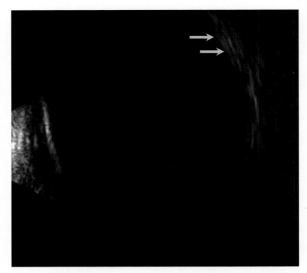

Fig. 33.2   B-scan ultrasonography of the lesion *(arrows),* a flat mass with medium acoustic solidity.

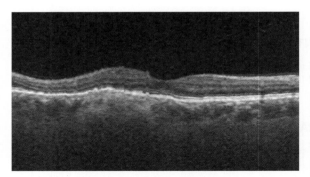

Fig. 33.3   Optical coherence tomography demonstrates the choroidal nevus, compressing the inner choroidal tissue. Note the shallow subretinal fluid with retracted photoreceptor morphology.

FOLLOW-UP

- At 4 months of follow-up, SRF on OCT was completely regressed, and her visual acuity had returned to 20/20.

KEY POINTS

- In a retrospective study of 3806 choroidal nevus patients, OCT showed SRF in 312 (9%).
- In multivariate analysis of factors at initial presentation predictive of growth into melanoma in 2211 eyes of 2075 patients, the most important factors for transformation into melanoma included SRF on OCT (hazard ratio, 3.11; 95% confidence interval (1.94–4.99), $P < 0.0001$).
- The prognosis for these patients is generally good. Management of choroidal nevus with SRF depends on visual symptoms, tumor size and location, presence, and amount of SRF. Options include observation, anti-VEGF injections, and laser photocoagulation.

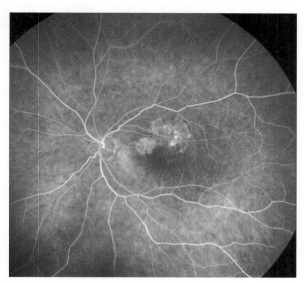

Fig. 33.4 Fluorescein angiogram of the lesion in venous phase showing hyperfluorescence of the lesion and multiple foci of hyperfluorescence temporally representing leakage points.

CHAPTER 34

Choroid Nevus With Pigment Epithelial Detachment

Caitlin Kelley-Smith ■ Aparna Ramasubramanian

Decreased Visual Acuity in a 58-Year-Old Female

HISTORY OF PRESENT ILLNESS

A previously healthy 58-year-old female presents with progressive blurring of vision right eye (OD). She was seen by an optometrist, was found to have a pigmented fundus lesion, and was referred to the ocular oncology service.

Exam

	OD	OS
Visual acuity	20/200	20/20
IOP (mm Hg)	16	15
Sclera/conjunctiva	White and quiet	White and quiet
Cornea	Clear	Clear
AC	Deep and quiet	Deep and quiet
Iris	Hazel iris, pupil round	Hazel iris, pupil round
Lens	Clear	Clear
Anterior vitreous	Clear	Clear
Retina/optic nerve	Normal optic nerve, pigmented choroidal lesion superotemporal to the macula, 3DD in diameter with multiple drusen, SRF, and no orange pigment (Fig. 34.1A)	Normal optic nerve, posterior and peripheral retina

3DD, 3 Disc diameters; *AC,* anterior chamber; *IOP,* intraocular pressure; *SRF,* subretinal fluid.

QUESTIONS TO ASK

- Have you had previous eye examinations?
- Do you have any family or personal history of melanoma or other cancers?

The patient has never had any previous eye examinations and was not aware of lesions in the fundus. She does not have any family history of melanoma. She denies any other significant past medical history.

No financial interest associated with the manuscript. No funding supports.

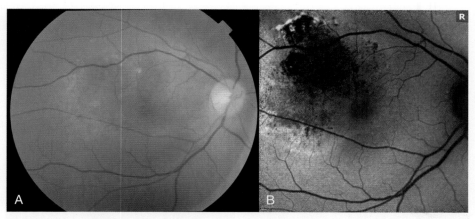

Fig. 34.1 (A) Fundus photograph showing the pigmented choroid nevus superotemporal to the macula with multiple drusen and subretinal fluid. (B) Autofluorescence shows predominant hypoautofluorescence corresponding to the choroid nevus and mild hyperautofluorescence in the region of subretinal fluid.

ASSESSMENT

- Pigmented choroidal lesion with SRF involving the macula

DIFFERENTIAL DIAGNOSIS

- Choroidal nevus
- Choroidal melanoma
- Choroidal metastasis
- Polypoidal choroidal vasculopathy

WORKING DIAGNOSIS

- Choroidal nevus with SRF, OD

INVESTIGATION AND TESTING

- B-scan ultrasound of OD showed echodense choroidal lesions measuring 2.7 mm in thickness.
- Autofluorescence showed no hyperfluorescent spots suggestive of orange pigment. There was faint hyperautofluorescence from the SRF (Fig. 34.1B).
- Optical coherence tomography showed the pigment epithelial detachment and surrounding SRF in the macular region (Fig. 34.2).

MANAGEMENT

- Patient underwent foveal sparing transpupillary thermotherapy and three intravitreal injections of bevacizumab (Avastin).

FOLLOW-UP

- The SRF improved following the intravitreal bevacizumab and transpupillary thermotherapy (Fig. 34.3). The patient's visual acuity improved to 20/70. The patient is on follow-up every 6 months, and after 4 years there is no growth of the choroid nevus.

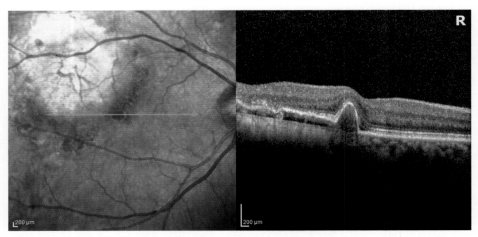

Fig. 34.2 Optical coherence tomography shows pigment epithelial detachment with subretinal fluid in the fovea.

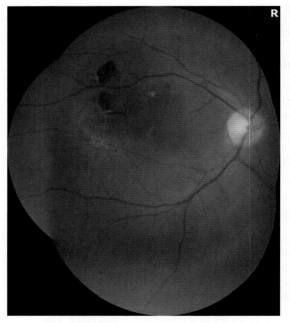

Fig. 34.3 Follow-up fundus photography showing scarring from the thermotherapy with resolved subretinal fluid.

KEY POINTS

- Choroid nevi are the most common primary intraocular tumors and arise from pigmented cells in the vascular choroid layer beneath the retina.
- Most choroid nevi are benign and do not affect visual acuity. Choroid nevi associated with increased thickness (>2 mm), SRF, and orange pigment are high risk for malignant choroidal melanomas.

- PED in a choroid nevus is not a risk factor for malignant transformation but can cause visual loss especially if the location is subfoveal.
- Choroid nevi can harbor a choroidal neovascular membrane under the PED, and that can be diagnosed by fluorescein angiography.
- Diagnostic tests such as ultrasound, fundus autofluorescence photography, and optical coherence tomography can be used to assess nevi growth or adverse clinical features.
- Choroid nevi with PED and SRF can be treated with anti-VEGF agents and laser to improve vision.
- A standard choroid nevus does not require any management and only needs to be evaluated once a year. Nevi associated with overlying PED or other clinical risk factors need to be evaluated every 4 to 6 months.

CHAPTER 35

Choroid Melanoma—Small

Jared Ching ■ Mandeep Sagoo

A Pigmented Choroidal Lesion With Suspicious Features

HISTORY OF PRESENT ILLNESS

A 67-year-old female was referred by her local optometrist to the Ocular Oncology Service at Moorfields Eye Hospital for a suspicious pigmented fundus lesion. The patient denied any visual symptoms and was otherwise fit and well with an unremarkable ocular history.

Exam

	OD	OS
Visual acuity	20/16	20/16
IOP (mm Hg)	20	21
Sclera/conjunctiva	White and quiet	White and quiet
Cornea	Clear	Clear
AC	Deep and quiet	Deep and quiet
Iris	Unremarkable	Unremarkable
Lens	Clear	Clear
Anterior vitreous	Clear	Clear
Retina/optic nerve	Normal optic disc, macular and peripheral retina	A melanocytic choroidal lesion temporal to the macula approximately 4 DDs with an associated shallow serous retinal detachment and scattered orange pigment Normal optic disc and peripheral retina (Fig. 35.1)

AC, Anterior chamber; *DD,* disc diameter; *IOP,* intraocular pressure.

QUESTIONS TO ASK

■ Have you had blurred vision, flashing lights, or floaters in your vision?
■ Have you ever been to the optometrist or ophthalmologist before and had photographs taken of the back of your eye?
■ Is there any history of cancer or abnormal skin moles in your family?

Visual symptoms including photopsias and floaters are absent in this case. The patient denies having any prior imaging. Her history is clear of any cancer diagnosis or atypical nevi in the family.

No financial interest associated with the manuscript. No funding supports.

156

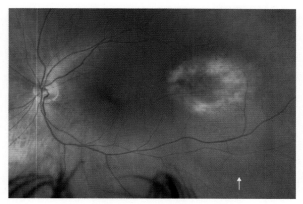

Fig. 35.1 Left eye showing pigmented choroidal lesion temporal to macula and inferior serous retinal detachment *(vertical arrow)*.

ASSESSMENT

- Pigmented choroidal lesion temporal to the macula, OS
- Orange pigment present within the pigmented lesion
- Serous detachment visible

DIFFERENTIAL DIAGNOSIS

- Benign choroidal nevus
- Suspicious choroidal nevus (indeterminate, requiring monitoring)
- Uveal melanoma
- Retinal pigment epithelial adenoma
- Subretinal hemorrhage secondary to age-related macular degeneration (if within macula) or peripheral exudative chorioretinopathy (if peripheral retina)
- Hamartoma of the retina and retinal pigment epithelium (RPE)
- Congenital hypertrophy of the RPE (CHRPE)
- Choroidal hemangioma

WORKING DIAGNOSIS

- Uveal melanoma

INVESTIGATION AND TESTING

- Fundus autofluorescence imaging demonstrates the gravitational serous retinal detachment characterized by the bright homogenous hyperautofluorescence inferior to the pigmented hypoautofluorescent choroidal lesion. Hyperautofluorescent dots within the tumor represent orange pigment (Fig. 35.2).
- Optical coherent tomography (OCT) confirms that the pigmented lesion is at the level of the choroid. Peritumoral and apical subretinal fluid (SRF) is present, and there is hyperreflective orange pigment on the surface of the RPE (Fig. 35.3).
- B-scan ultrasound confirmed the presence of an elevated choroidal lesion of medium echogenicity with associated SRF. Measurements were a transverse base of 6.1 mm, longitudinal base of 5.9 mm, and elevation of 1.5 mm. Blood flow studies by color flow mapping were not possible as the tumor was too shallow (Fig. 35.4).

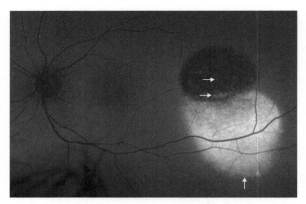

Fig. 35.2 Fundus autofluorescence demonstrating hyperautofluoroescent orange pigments *(horizontal white arrows)* and hyperautofluoroescent serous retinal detachment *(vertical arrow).*

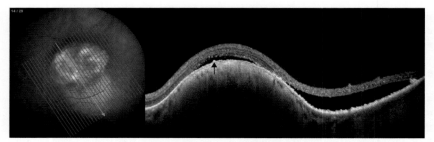

Fig. 35.3 Spectral domain optical coherence tomography demonstrating a lesion arising from the choroid with associated subretinal fluid and punctate hyperreflective dots overlying the retinal pigment epithelium representing orange pigment *(vertical arrow).*

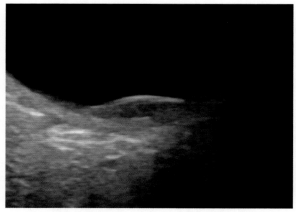

Fig. 35.4 B-scan ultrasound demonstrating choroidal lesion of medium echogenicity with associated subretinal fluid.

TABLE 35.1 ■ **TFSOM-DIM Imaging**

Variable	Letter	Mnemonic	Testing	Hazard Ratio (Mean) Multivariate Analysis	P Value
Thickness tumor >2 mm	T	To	US	3.80	< 0.0001
Fluid subretinal	F	Find	OCT	3.56	< 0.0001
					0.0003
Symptoms visual acuity <20/50	S	Small	Snellen VA	2.28	0.0050
Orange pigment	O	Ocular	AF	3.07	0.0004
Melanoma acoustic hollowness	M	Melanoma	US	2.10	0.0020
Diameter tumor > 5 mm	DIM	Doing IMaging	Photography	1.84	0.0275

The **To Find Small Ocular Melanoma Doing IMaging"** (TFSOM-DIM) mnemonic was developed by Shields and colleagues to determine the likelihood of transformation of a choroidal nevus into melanoma. The mean 5-year estimates for transformation into a uveal melanoma are 1% for those with no risk factors, 11% with one risk factor, 22% with two risk factors, 34% with three risk factors, 51% with four risk factors, and 55% with five risk factors.

MANAGEMENT

- Patient underwent ruthenium plaque brachytherapy.
- Systemic evaluation and surveillance were conducted.

FOLLOW-UP

- The patient had responded well to therapy at 6-month follow-up with no signs of local tumor recurrence. Systemic investigations, including liver imaging, revealed no metastatic involvement. She continued ocular and systemic surveillance.

KEY POINTS

- Uveal melanoma is the most common primary intraocular cancer in adults but is relatively rare, occurring in approximately 5 to 10 cases per million population per year.
- The diagnosis is clinical and aided by multimodality imaging, such as color fundus photography, autofluorescence, OCT, and ultrasound of the eye.
- Use of a mnemonic such as TFSMOM-DIM[1] (**To Find Small Ocular Melanoma Doing IMaging**; Table 35.1) or MOLES score[2] (Table 35.2) assists in diagnosing suspicious choroidal melanocytic lesions.
- Previously small suspicious melanocytic lesions were often observed for growth as a surrogate marker for malignancy.
- A European study found that small uveal melanomas with a basal diameter of more than 3 mm are able to metastasize.[3]
- Many centers are offering treatment earlier rather than waiting for documented growth.
- Management of small uveal melanomas requires treatment with local radiotherapy, such as plaque brachytherapy or proton beam radiotherapy, which has a high rate of local tumor control.
- The prognosis for these patients is dependent on whether metastasis occurs, which in turn is largely determined by the presence of genetic mutations such as BAP1 inactivation.

TABLE 35.2 ■ MOLES Scoring System

Risk Factor	Severity	Score
Mushroom shape	Absent	0
	Unsure/early growth through RPE	1
	Present, with overhang	2
Orange pigment	Absent	0
	Unsure/trace (i.e., dusting)	1
	Confluent clumps	2
Large size[a]	Thickness <1.0 mm ("flat/minimal thickening") and diameter <3 DD	0
	Thickness = 1.0 mm–2.0 mm ("subtle dome shape") and/or diameter = 3–4 DD	1
	Thickness >2.0 mm ("significant thickening") and/or diameter >4 DD	2
Enlargement[b]	No growth or no previous ophthalmoscopy	0
	Unsure growth/"new" lesion not documented after previous ophthalmoscopy	1
	Definite growth or new tumor confirmed with sequential imaging	2
Subretinal fluid	Absent	0
	Trace, if minimal and detected only with OCT	1
	Definite, seen without OCT, or extending beyond tumor margin	2
	Total score out of 10	/10
	Tumor category is based on score out of 10[c]	

DD, Disk diamater (= 1.5 mm); OCT, optical coherence tomography.

The MOLES scoring system was developed by Damato and colleagues to aid assessment of melanocytic choroidal lesions for non-experts. A total MOLES score of 0 warrants monitoring every 1–2 years by an optometrist; a score of 2 requires a non-urgent specialist assessment with multimodal imaging; and a score of 3 or more is strongly suggestive of a uveal melanoma necessitating an urgent referral to a specialist.[2]

[a]Ignore thickness if this cannot be measured.

[b]Assume enlargement has occurred if thickness is >3 mm or diameter is >5 DD, and give this a score of 2.

[c]Categorize tumors according to the total score: 0 = common nevus; 2 = high-risk nevus; and 3 or more = probable melanoma.

References

1. Shields CL, Lim LS, Dalvin LA, Shields JA. Small choroidal melanoma: Detection with multimodal imaging and management with plaque radiotherapy or AU-011 nanoparticle therapy. *Curr Opin Ophthalmol.* 2019;30(3):206–214. doi:10.1097/ICU.0000000000000560.
2. Roelofs KA, O'Day R, Harby LA, et al. The MOLES system for planning management of melanocytic choroidal tumors: Is it safe? *Cancers (Basel).* 2020;12(5):1311. doi:10.3390/cancers12051311.
3. Jouhi S, Jager MJ, de Geus SJR, et al. The Small Fatal Choroidal Melanoma Study: A survey by the European Ophthalmic Oncology Group. *Am J Ophthalmol.* 2019;202:100–108. doi:10.1016/j.ajo.2019.01.031.

CHAPTER 36

Choroid Melanoma—Medium

Ethan Willis ■ David Reichstein ■ Anderson Brock

Ongoing Photopsia in a 49-Year-Old Woman

HISTORY OF PRESENT ILLNESS

A 49-year-old female presents with left eye photopsia. She complained of ongoing flashes of light in the left eye for 6–9 months prior to presentation. She had no prior ocular history or trauma to either eye.

Exam

	OD	OS
Visual acuity	Sc 20/30	Sc 20/40
	PH 20/20	PH 20/25
IOP (mm HG)	18	17
Sclera/conjunctiva	White and quiet	White and quiet
Cornea	Clear	Clear
AC	Deep and quiet	Deep and quiet
Iris	Flat	Flat
	No rubeosis	No rubeosis
	Within normal limits	Within normal limits
Lens	1+ NS	1+ NS
Anterior vitreous	Clear	Clear
Retina/optic nerve	Normal optic nerve, posterior and peripheral retina	Elevated pigmented choroidal lesion (9 mm x 9 mm x mm) with overlying SRF and orange pigment (0 mm from optic nerve, 3 mm from fovea) (Fig. 36.1)

AC, Anterior chamber; *IOP,* intraocular pressure; *NS,* nuclear sclerosis; *PH,* pinhole; *SC,* without correction; *SRF,* subretinal fluid.

QUESTIONS TO ASK

- Have you noticed any new flashes or floaters in your vision?
- Have you had any recent changes in visual acuity?
- Do you have any history of cancer?

The patient had an increase in flashes in her left eye for 6–9 months prior to presentation. She denied any significant changes in visual acuity. No history of cancer was noted.

No financial interest associated with the manuscript. No funding supports.

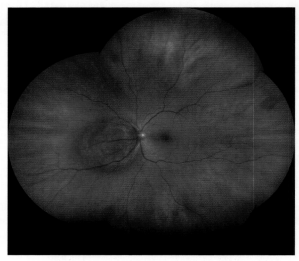

Fig. 36.1   Left eye showing an elevated mass bordering the optic nerve extending into the vitreous cavity.

ASSESSMENT

- Pigmented choroidal mass, OS
- Serous retinal detachment, OS

DIFFERENTIAL DIAGNOSIS

- Choroidal melanoma
- Choroidal hemangioma
- Pigmented choroidal neovascular membrane
- Choroidal nevus

WORKING DIAGNOSIS

- Choroidal melanoma with serous retinal detachment, OS

INVESTIGATION AND TESTING

- B-scan ultrasound of OS showed a mass arising from the choroid extending 4.8 mm into the vitreous cavity (Fig. 36.2).
- Optical coherence tomography (OCT) showed an elevated mass with overlying subretinal fluid (SRF) (Fig. 36.3).
- Autofluorescence photos showed a choroidal lesion with hyperautofluorescence consistent with orange pigment (Fig. 36.4).
- Intraocular lesion was evaluated for concerning features of malignancy, including orange pigmentation, ultrasonographic hollowness, subretinal fluid, elevation, and absence of drusen.

MANAGEMENT

- The patient initially underwent radiation via plaque brachytherapy of OS with 85 Gy delivered to the tumor apex.

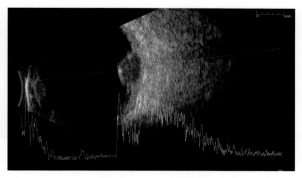

Fig. 36.2   Ultrasound showing a mass extending from the choroid into the vitreous cavity.

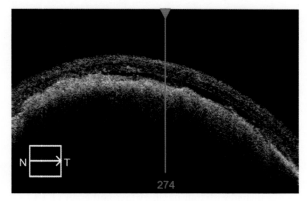

Fig. 36.3   Optical coherence tomography showing an elevated choroidal mass with overlying subretinal fluid.

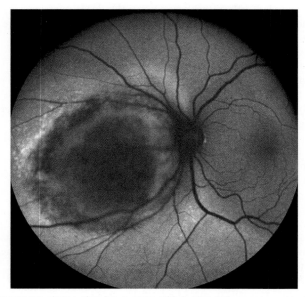

Fig. 36.4   Autofluorescence photos showing a mass with hyperautofluorescence consistent with orange pigment.

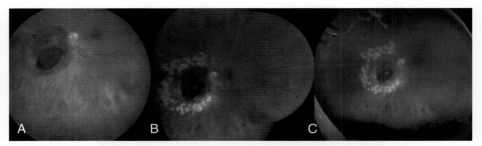

Fig. 36.5 Fundus photos showing regression of the melanoma at different intervals following radiation therapy: (A) 4 months, (B) 8 months, and (C) 17 months.

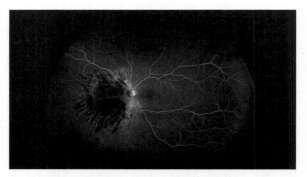

Fig. 36.6 Fluorescein angiography showing multiple branch retinal vein occlusions on the lesion.

- The melanoma was treated with transpupillary thermotherapy (TTT) 4 months after radiation therapy.
- Genetic testing via Castle Biosciences DecisionDx-UM gene expression profile (GEP), PRAME, and next-generation sequencing panel for uveal melanoma were performed.

FOLLOW-UP

- Following plaque brachytherapy and TTT, the melanoma has remained regressed on follow-up for 18 months (Fig. 36.5).
- The DecisionDx-UM genetic testing indicated a class 1A, PRAME-negative tumor with clinically significant alterations in the *GNA11* and *EIF1AX* genes.
- The patient developed multiple branch retinal vein occlusions (BRVOs) (Fig. 36.6) secondary to radiation retinopathy 17 months after radiation therapy and was treated with panretinal photocoagulation (PRP).
- The patient is set to follow up in clinic 4 months after PRP treatment.

KEY POINTS

- Choroidal melanoma is a common intraocular malignancy, and its metastases can be deadly.
- The prognosis for patients with choroidal melanoma is generally good if the tumor is treated prior to systemic metastasis.
- GEP/PRAME/Seq testing for uveal melanoma allows for risk-specific surveillance and management for metastatic disease (Table 36.1).

TABLE 36.1 ■ Castle Bioscience's Description of DecisionDx-UM Results Based on Molecular Signature Class

Molecular Signature Class	Percentage Metastasis Free at 3 Years	Percentage Metastasis Free at 5 Years
Class 1A	98%	98%
Class 1B	93%	79%
Class 2	50%	28%

$n = 514$; Log-rank (Mantel-Cox) test; $p < 0.0001$.
Clinical Experience for Classes 1A, 1B, and 2.
The DecisionDx-UM assay has been evaluated in over 1300 patients with uveal melanoma to date, including those from a prospective, multicenter study to validate the predictive accuracy of the gene expression–based molecular assay. Outcomes were collected, and the ability of the molecular signature to predict metastasis was evaluated. The most recent censor date of the prospective study (June 9, 2011) included 514 patients with follow-up data available for analysis. The following are the outcomes for metastasis of the predicted low-risk (class 1A), intermediate-risk (class 1B), and high-risk (class 2) molecular signatures.

- PRAME may increase the time to metastasis in class 2 patients and may increase the likelihood of metastasis in class 1 patients.
- PRAME positivity in class 1 and 2 tumors was not significantly correlated with monosomy 3.
- PRAME positivity was associated with *BAP1* mutations, likely because *BAP1* mutations are most prevalent in class 2 patients.

CHAPTER 37

Choroid Melanoma—Large

Aneesha Ahluwalia ■ Chaow Charoenkijkajorn ■ Prithvi Mruthyunjaya

Painless Visual Field Deficit and Photopsias in a 72-Year-Old Male

HISTORY OF PRESENT ILLNESS

A 72-year-old White male with a history of hypertension presents with a temporal blind spot in his right eye that developed over the past few weeks and several months of intermittent flashes of light in his right eye. He denies any ocular pain. His ocular history is notable for cataracts in both eyes.

Exam

	OD	OS
Visual acuity	20/70–20/30 ph	20/70–20/30 ph
IOP (mm Hg)	11	12
Sclera/conjunctiva	White and quiet	White and quiet
Cornea	Clear	Clear
AC	Deep and quiet	Deep and quiet
Iris	Round and reactive	Round and reactive
Lens	2+ nuclear sclerotic cataract	2+ nuclear sclerotic cataract
Anterior vitreous	Clumps of orange pigment in the vitreous overlying a mass	Clear
Retina/optic nerve	Large hyperpigmented choroidal lesion approximately 11 mm × 11 mm in base with overlying orange pigment and surface vascularity; lesion overhangs the optic nerve head and extends from the nasal midperiphery to 5 mm from the fovea; the optic nerve is not visible; no subretinal fluid (Fig. 37.1)	Normal optic nerve, macula, and peripheral retina

AC, Anterior chamber; *IOP*, intraocular pressure; *ph*, pinhole.

QUESTIONS TO ASK

■ Do you or anyone in your family have a history of cancer?
■ Has anyone told you that you have a mole or freckle in the back of your eye?
■ Do you have any history of ocular trauma or ocular surgery?
■ Have you had any systemic symptoms like weight loss or abdominal pain?

No financial interests are associated with the manuscript. Funding: Research to Prevent Blindness, NEI P30-026877, Irene and Alan Adler Ocular Oncology Initiative.

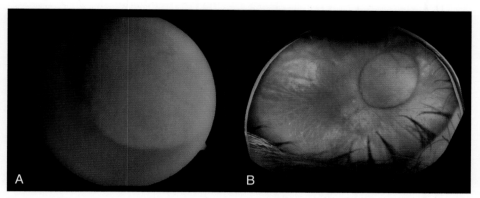

Fig. 37.1 (A) Color fundus photograph of the right eye and (B) ultra-wide field imaging demonstrating a large, round, elevated choroidal lesion obscuring the optic nerve. The surface of the lesion is vascularized with overlying scattered orange pigment.

The patient reports no personal or family history of cancer. He cannot recall his most recent dilated eye examination and has never been told that he has any intraocular pathology apart from cataracts. He denies any history of ocular surgery or trauma. He denies any systemic symptoms.

ASSESSMENT

- Elevated, dome-shaped, pigmented choroidal mass, OD
- Vitreous pigment, OD

DIFFERENTIAL DIAGNOSIS

- Choroidal melanoma
- Choroidal nevus
- Choroidal metastasis

WORKING DIAGNOSIS

- Choroidal melanoma, OD

INVESTIGATION AND TESTING

- B-scan ultrasound demonstrated a mushroom-shaped, elevated choroidal lesion measuring 11.9 mm × 10.7 mm × 9.2 mm overhanging the optic nerve (Fig. 37.2A).
- A-scan ultrasound demonstrated initially medium then progressive low internal reflectivity with intravascular pulsations (Fig. 37.2B).
- Optical coherence tomograph (OCT) through the lesion was limited by tumor thickness but showed an elevated mass with surface hyperreflectivity and an absence of subretinal fluid.
- Intravenous fluorescein angiography (IVFA) demonstrated early filling of the choroidal tumor with a dual circulation pattern and late leakage with overlying hyperfluorescent patches.
- CT chest, abdomen, and pelvis with contrast did not demonstrate any evidence of extraocular malignancy.

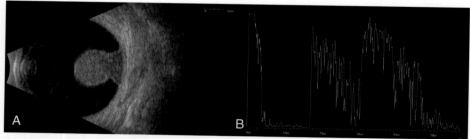

Fig. 37.2 (A) B-scan ultrasonography showing a mushroom-shaped choroidal lesion measuring 11.9 mm × 10.7 mm × 9.2 mm. (B) A-scan ultrasonography of the same lesion demonstrating initially medium-low, then progressive low internal reflectivity with intravascular pulsations.

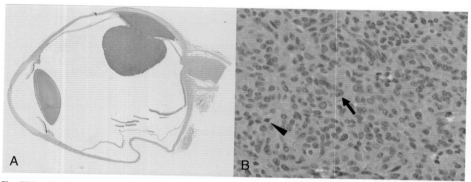

Fig. 37.3 (A) Oblique globe section demonstrating a large mushroom-shaped choroidal mass erupting through Bruch's membrane. (B) On microscopic examination, the choroidal mass is composed predominantly of round cells with abundant cytoplasm, large nuclei, and prominent nucleoli, consistent with an epithelioid morphology *(arrow)*. There is also scattered pigment *(arrowhead)*.

MANAGEMENT

- Discussed with the patient potential treatment options of plaque brachytherapy versus proton beam radiation versus enucleation. Given the large size of the tumor and the ensuing risk of radiation toxicity, it was recommended he undergo enucleation.
- The patient underwent enucleation with placement of an orbital implant.
- At the time of enucleation, a fresh tumor sample was extracted with fine-needle aspiration (FNA).
- Histopathology revealed a large, mushroom-shaped mass composed of epithelioid cells with scattered melanin pigment arising from the choroid with invasion of Bruch's membrane (Fig. 37.3A–B). There was no evidence of extrascleral extension of the mass or postlaminar optic nerve invasion.
- Immunohistochemical staining was positive for the melanocyte molecular markers: *HMB-45* and *Melan-A. BAP1 (BRCA1*-associated protein-1) nuclear staining was expressed throughout the tumor, and the mass was preferentially expressed antigen in melanoma (*PRAME*) negative.
- The overall gene expression profile was consistent with a class 1A tumor, predictive of low future risk of metastatic disease.

FOLLOW-UP

The patient has remained stable for 3 years without evidence of recurrent disease. He receives annual liver imaging, liver function tests, and chest imaging for metastatic surveillance.

KEY POINTS

- Choroidal melanomas are the most common primary intraocular malignancy.
- Known risk factors for choroidal melanoma include light skin color, light iris color, welding exposure, and northern European ancestry.
- Like other uveal melanomas, choroidal melanomas are primarily composed of a mixture of three cell types: spindle A, spindle B, and epithelioid. The epithelioid morphology is associated with the greatest metastatic potential and mortality. The spindle morphology has the best prognosis, and tumors consisting of a mixture of spindle and epithelioid cells have an intermediate prognosis.
- When confined to the uvea, choroidal melanomas are often small and disc shaped. An enlarging tumor can rupture through Bruch's membrane, acquiring a characteristic collar-button or mushroom morphology.
- Tumors overhanging or involving the optic disc can be treated with radiation therapy, although the risk of radiation-associated complications must be considered.
- Choroidal melanomas rarely present with metastatic disease, but all patients should undergo systemic evaluation with dedicated chest and abdominal imaging (CT or MRI is preferred).
- *PRAME* is an antigen biomarker that is associated with a nearly 10 times higher risk of metastatic disease in patients with uveal melanomas. Loss of the *BAP1* gene has also been implicated as a risk factor for worse prognosis. Currently, genetic testing is recommended as a supplementary, rather than primary, prognostic factor.
- For large choroidal melanomas (>10 mm in thickness or 16 mm in basal dimension), enucleation is the preferred treatment. Increased tumor thickness is associated with higher recurrence rates and increased risk of vision- and globe-threatening radiation-associated complications.
- After therapy, the incidence of metastatic disease at 25 years can be as high as 50%. The liver is the primary site of metastasis, followed by the lungs, skin, and bone. Larger tumor size is a predictor of eventual metastatic disease independent of primary tumor control. Therefore, all patients with large choroidal melanomas are advised to undergo routine systemic surveillance. Genetic risk profiling can guide the frequency of testing. A medical oncologist may be consulted to manage systemic screening and treatment of metastatic disease.

CHAPTER 38

Choroid Melanoma—Extrascleral Extension

Sarah Brumley ■ Dan S. Gombos

Choroidal Lesion and Corectopia in a 68-Year-Old Female

HISTORY OF PRESENT ILLNESS

A 68-year-old female with no prior cancer history presents with a choroidal neoplasm of the right eye. Patient states that the lesion was discovered during her previous cataract surgery, and it has progressed, now protruding through the iris. Right eye is achy and throbs. She has no prior significant ocular history to either eye.

Exam

	OD	OS
Visual acuity	Counting fingers	20/50
IOP (mm Hg)	12	13
Sclera/conjunctiva	2.4-mm × 2.6-mm dark lesion protruding through sclera inferior to cornea	White and quiet
Cornea	Few keratic precipitates inferiorly	Clear
AC	Shallow	Deep and quiet
Iris	2.4-mm × 4.4-mm inferior scalloped brown lesion with neovascularization, iris pushed upward from mass, lesions protruding through pupil	Round and reactive
Lens	Pigment on lens	2+ cortical cataract
Anterior vitreous	No view	No cells
Retina/optic nerve	No view	Normal, 0.25 C/D, reticular changes in RPE periphery

AC, Anterior chamber; *C/D,* cup to disc ratio; *IOP,* intraocular pressure; *RPE,* retinal pigment epithelium.

QUESTIONS TO ASK

- Have you experienced pain in the right eye?
- Have you experienced flashes of light in the right eye?
- Any history of an ocular spot or birthmark?
- Is there any history of cancer in the family?
- Is there any other relevant past medical history?

No financial interest associated with the manuscript. No funding supports.

The patient has never complained of pain or flashing lights in either eye. No signs of redness in each eye (OU). Patient denies history of cancer in the family, but she reports smoking 1.5 packs/day for 60 years.

ASSESSMENT

- Malignant melanoma of right choroid: stage IIIB, T4c, N0, M0
- Malignant neoplasm of overlapping sites, OD

DIFFERENTIAL DIAGNOSIS

- Iris nevus
- Choroidal nevus
- Medulloepithelioma
- Leiomyoma/leiomyosarcoma
- Choroidal hemangioma
- Peripheral exudative hemorrhagic chorioretinopathy

WORKING DIAGNOSIS

- Uveal melanoma with extraocular extension, OD

INVESTIGATION AND TESTING

- B-scan ultrasound, OD, showed a large mass with basal dimensions of 12.3 mm × 16.4 mm and apical dimension of 16.5 mm.
- Ultrasound biomicroscopy (UBM)/anterior segment OD showed a mass located on the iris, ciliary body with overlying conjunctival mass, and pars plana with medium internal reflectivity (Fig. 38.3).
- MRI of brain and orbits with contrast showed 15 mm × 25 mm × 14 mm mass without posterior orbital extension; no intracranial metastasis (Fig. 38.1).

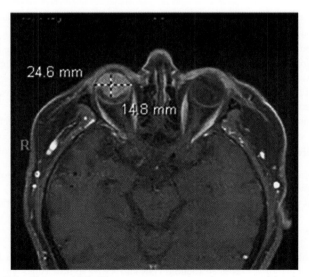

Fig. 38.1   Right eye MRI without contrast showing a large mass of the choroid.

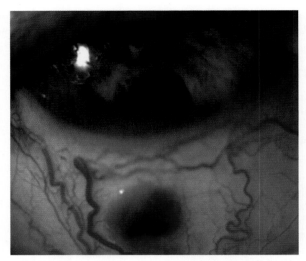

Fig. 38.2   External photo demonstrating extraocular extension.

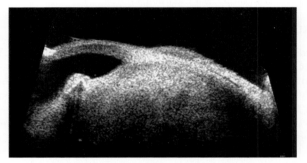

Fig. 38.3   Ultrasound biomicroscopy showing intraocular neoplasm with extraocular extension.

- CT of chest, abdomen, and pelvis with contrast showed an indeterminate 6-mm nodule in the lower lobe of the right lung, as well as two hypoattenuating foci on the liver.
- Fundus photos, OD, showed a large pigmented mass.
- Slit-lamp photography, OD, showed a pigmented mass, with concern for extrascleral extension of intraocular tumor (Fig. 38.2).
- A PET scan showed no local hypermetabolism and no regional lymphadenopathy.

MANAGEMENT

- The potential management and treatment options discussed included proton beam radiation therapy, plaque brachytherapy, and modified enucleation.
- The patient underwent prognostic biopsy and enucleation, OD, with insertion of an implant.

FOLLOW-UP

- Histopathology revealed a large mass arising from the ciliary body and iris that displayed mixed cell melanoma (>10% epithelioid cells and <90% spindle cells) with involvement of the sclera, choroid, ciliary body, iris, Schlemm's canal, and anterior extrascleral extension.

- The patient was offered additional radiotherapy to the orbit but elected not to proceed.
- Genetic testing showed a class 2 molecular signature with discriminant value of 0.91 and *PRAME* positivity, indicating a high risk (72%) of clinical metastasis in 5 years, and mutations at the *GNA11* and *BAP1* genes.

KEY POINTS

- Uveal melanomas are rare tumors of the choroid that develop from melanocytes in the highly pigmented uveal tract. They account for just 5% of all melanoma but comprise the most common eye cancer.
- Extraocular extension beyond the globe increases the staging and decreases the prognosis.
- Uveal melanoma has a known association with *BRCA1*-associated protein 1 mutations and G-protein subunit alpha Q mutations.
- Management of advanced uveal melanoma with extraocular extension is best treated with a modified enucleation. Some prefer to insert nonintegrated implants in such cases and administer postenucleation radiation therapy. Proton beam radiotherapy has been successfully used in select cases.
- The prognosis for these patients is generally good if the tumor stays confined to the globe.

CHAPTER 39

Choroid Melanoma—Isolated Liver Metastasis

Emine Kilic ■ Janelle Marie Fassbender Adeniran ■ Aparna Ramasubramanian

Incidental Finding on Routine Eye Screening

HISTORY OF PRESENT ILLNESS

A previously healthy 62-year-old female was seen by an optometrist and was found to have a pigmented fundus lesion and was referred to the ocular oncology service. She noted no changes in her vision.

Exam

	OD	OS
Visual acuity	20/20	20/20
IOP (mm Hg)	16	15
Sclera/conjunctiva	White and quiet	White and quiet
Cornea	Clear	Clear
AC	Deep and quiet	Deep and quiet
Iris	Hazel iris, pupil round	Hazel iris, pupil round
Lens	1+ nuclear sclerosis	1+ nuclear sclerosis
Anterior vitreous	Clear	Clear
Retina/optic nerve	Normal optic nerve, posterior and peripheral retina	Normal optic nerve, normal macula; pigmented elevated choroidal lesion inferotemporally measuring 14 mm × 12 mm with surrounding subretinal fluid and overlying orange pigment (Fig. 39.1)

AC, Anterior chamber; *IOP,* intraocular pressure.

QUESTIONS TO ASK

- Have you had previous eye examinations?
- Do you have any personal or family history of melanoma?
- Do you have any history of cancer?

The patient has never had any previous eye examinations and was not aware of lesions in the fundus. She does not have any family history of melanoma. She denies any other significant medical history.

No financial interest associated with the manuscript. No funding supports.

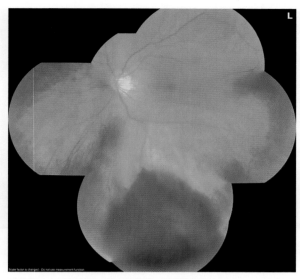

Fig. 39.1 Pigmented elevated choroidal lesion inferotemporally with surrounding subretinal fluid and overlying orange pigment.

ASSESSMENT

- Pigmented elevated choroidal lesion with subretinal fluid (SRF) and orange pigment

DIFFERENTIAL DIAGNOSIS

- Choroidal nevus
- Choroidal melanoma
- Choroidal metastasis
- Peripheral exudative hemorrhagic chorioretinopathy

WORKING DIAGNOSIS

- Choroidal melanoma OS

INVESTIGATION AND TESTING

- B-scan ultrasound of OS showed choroidal lesion with acoustic hollowness measuring 4.8-mm thickness.
- Optical coherence tomography (OCT) showed elevated choroidal lesion with SRF (Fig. 39.2).
- Fluorescein angiography showed early filling of the choroidal lesion with late leakage.
- CT chest and MRI abdomen did not show any evidence of metastatic disease.

MANAGEMENT

- Patient underwent plaque brachytherapy with I-125. Additional transpupillary thermotherapy was performed after the SRF resolved.

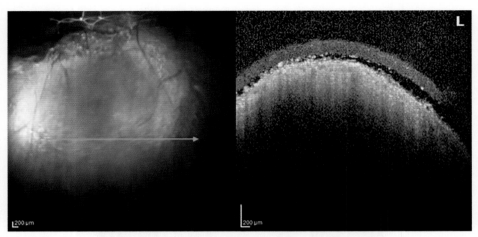

Fig. 39.2 Optical coherence tomography showing on left side the location of the lesion on the fundus *(green arrow)* and right image shows an elevated choroidal lesion with surrounding subretinal fluid (SRF).

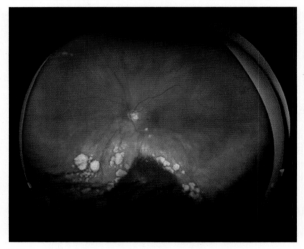

Fig. 39.3 The choroidal tumor after plaque radiotherapy showing a good response and a decreased thickness.

- Gene expression profiling at the time of plaque placement showed class 2 tumor with high risk for metastatic disease.
- Patient elected close monitoring without any prophylactic treatment.

FOLLOW-UP

- The choroidal tumor showed a good response and decreased to a thickness of 2.8 mm (Fig. 39.3). Sector panretinal photocoagulation and antivascular endothelial growth factor (anti-VEGF) injections were done for controlling radiation retinopathy. The patient's visual acuity was 20/40 OS.
- The patient has chest and abdomen imaging every 4 months.

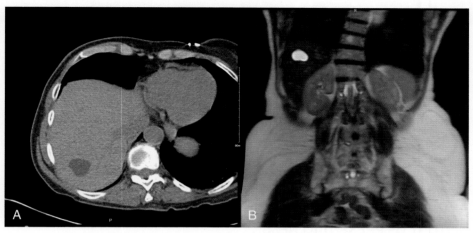

Fig. 39.4   (A) Confirmation of the solitary liver metastasis on CT and (B) on MRI.

- She was noted to have an isolated liver metastasis during routine monitoring at 5 years following primary treatment of the choroidal melanoma. The isolated liver metastasis was confirmed on CT (Fig. 39.4A) and MRI (Fig. 39.4B). She underwent stereotactic radiation to the liver metastasis with good response and no other detected sites of metastasis.

KEY POINTS

- Intraocular choroidal melanoma is the most common primary intraocular tumor in adults.
- Metastatic disease occurs in approximately 50% of patients over the first 10 years.
- The liver is involved in 90% of patients with metastatic disease.
- The prognosis is related to the genetic makeup of the primary melanoma, where a *BAP1* or *SF3B1* mutation, or a class 1B or class 2 expression profile, is associated with a higher metastatic risk.
- Screening at diagnosis is imperative as 2% of the patients will have disseminated disease at diagnosis.
- Despite treatment, for patients with liver metastasis, the mortality is 80% at 1 year, 92% at 2 years, and only 1% surviving over 5 years.
- The treatment options for isolated liver metastasis include surgical resection, transarterial embolization, selective internal radiotherapy, isolated hepatic perfusion (IHP), hepatic artery infusion, and immunoembolization.

CHAPTER 40

Choroid Melanoma—Diffuse Metastasis

Rachel Curtis ■ Ezekiel Weis

Retinal Detachment and 1 Month of Decreased Visual Acuity in a 64-Year-Old White Female

HISTORY OF PRESENT ILLNESS

A previously healthy 64-year-old female presents to her family physician with 1 month of gradual-onset blurred vision in the left eye. She is sent to an optometrist for an eye exam and is diagnosed with a detached retina. Upon urgent referral to the retina service, a choroidal lesion with high suspicion for melanoma is recognized. The patient is seen by the ocular oncology service the following day.

Exam

	OD	OS
Visual acuity	20/20-2	20/50 (no improvement with pinhole)
IOP (mm Hg)	15	15
Anterior segment	No ocular melanocytosis	No ocular melanocytosis, no sentinel vessels
	Phakic, 2+ NS	Phakic, 2+ NS
Posterior segment	Normal optic nerve, unremarkable macula and peripheral retina	Superior, elevated pigmented choroidal mass with associated subretinal fluid
		16-mm radial dimension x 12-mm circumferential dimension
		0.5 mm from the optic nerve head and 2 mm from the fovea

IOP, Intraocular pressure; *NS,* nuclear sclerotic cataract.

QUESTIONS TO ASK

■ Do you have any personal history of cancer?
■ Do you have any family history of cancer?
■ Do you have any past ocular history, including history of choroidal nevus?

The patient denies any personal or family history of cancer. There is no prior documentation of any ocular disease, intraocular lesion, or nevi.

No financial interest associated with the manuscript. No funding supports.

ASSESSMENT

Pigmented elevated choroidal lesion with subretinal fluid

DIFFERENTIAL DIAGNOSIS

- Choroidal melanoma
- Choroidal nevus
- Metastasis
- Retinal hemorrhage
- Choroidal hemangioma
- Congenital hypertrophy of the retinal pigment epithelium (CHRPE)
- Peripheral exudative hemorrhagic chorioretinopathy (PEHCR)

WORKING DIAGNOSIS

- Choroidal melanoma

INVESTIGATION AND TESTING

The tests in Table 40.1 should be ordered on every patient when choroidal melanoma is suspected.

Other testing that may be helpful in further differentiating choroidal melanoma from other "pseudomelanomas" may include the following:

- Fundus autofluorescence
- Optical coherence tomography (OCT)-angiography
- Fluorescein and/or indocyanine green angiography

Management: This pigmented choroidal lesion exhibits all of the characteristics of a choroidal melanoma requiring treatment. The following was discussed with the patient:

- The option of either enucleation or plaque radiotherapy. Specifically, it was emphasized that the mortality rates are identical regardless of treatment choice, but local plaque radiotherapy is intended to treat the choroidal melanoma with the intent of preserving the globe.
- Significant vision loss directly related to the plaque radiotherapy, especially given the size and location of the melanoma.

TABLE 40.1 ■ **Test for Suspected Choroidal Melanoma**

Diagnostic Procedure	Result in This Patient	Corresponding Figure
Fundus photography	As described above	Fig. 40.1
A and B scan ultrasound	Dome shaped, acoustically hollow lesion, with adjacent subretinal fluid	Fig. 40.2
	Internal reflectivity followed a decrescendo pattern	
	Ultrasound height 6.91 mm	
	Intralesional vascularity noted	
OCT macula	Subretinal fluid with a CFT of 386 μm with shaggy photoreceptors noted	Fig. 40.3A
OCT through the choroidal lesion	Subretinal and intraretinal fluid	Fig. 40.3B

CFT, Central foveal thickness; *OCT,* optical coherence tomography.

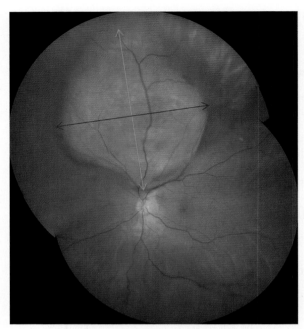

Fig. 40.1 Fundus photograph demonstrating an elevated pigmented mass superior to the optic nerve in the left eye. The *green line* represents the radial dimension of the lesion as measured with a 20D lens, and the *blue line* represents the circumferential dimension.

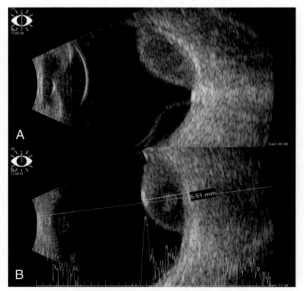

Fig. 40.2 B-scan ultrasound demonstrating (A) a dome-shaped acoustically hollow lesion arising from the choroid with adjacent retinal detachment and (B) measurements of the lesion measuring 6.91 mm in thickness with (A) scan overlay.

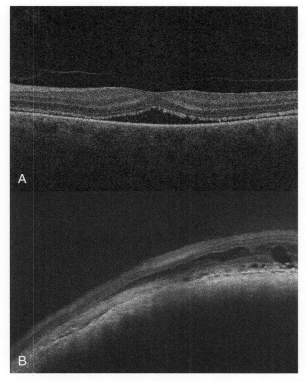

Fig. 40.3 OCT images of the left eye demonstrating (A) subretinal fluid in the macula and (B) small amounts of subretinal fluid associated with the lesion as well as intraretinal fluid.

- The natural history of choroidal melanoma, including the risk of metastasis (most commonly affecting the liver), and the need for regular imaging surveillance regardless of local treatment.
- Molecular testing and GEP were offered to the patient in the form of FNAB of the choroidal melanoma to be completed at the time of plaque insertion for further characterization of the lesion and expanded prognostic information.

LOCAL TREATMENT

- Conformal plaque brachytherapy utilizing I-125 was successfully performed with a 5-day insertion time. GEP showed a class 2 *PRAME*-negative result.
- At the time of treatment, metastatic workup was conducted, including complete blood count (CBC) and liver function tests, which were unremarkable, as well as posteroanterior (PA) and lateral chest x-rays and whole-body PET/CT that showed no evidence of metastatic disease.

FOLLOW-UP

- The patient was seen at regular intervals after plaque brachytherapy to follow evidence of tumor regression and appropriate healing, starting at 1 month postprocedure (Fig. 40.4).

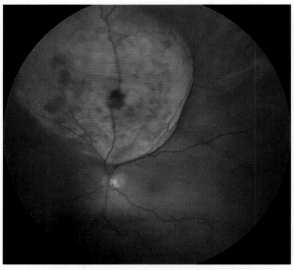

Fig. 40.4 Fundus photograph of the left eye 1 month post–plaque brachytherapy treatment with resolving overlying retinal hemorrhages from fine needle aspiration biopsy (FNAB).

- Signs of local treatment success include the following:
  - Retinal atrophy surrounding the tumor site
  - Resolution of subretinal fluid
  - Resolution of orange pigment (if present)
  - Decreased tumor thickness and increased acoustic solidity on B-scan ultrasound
- Excellent local tumor response to plaque brachytherapy was achieved (Fig. 40.5).
- Regular screening for metastasis was conducted, including interval abdominal ultrasound (MRI abdomen or PET/CT scans at defined intervals).
- Unfortunately, 16 months following the choroidal melanoma diagnosis, a 2.5-cm hypervascular mass was detected on MRI in the inferior aspect of the liver (segment 6), with numerous other foci of arterial hypervascularity suggestive of multiple (diffuse) hepatic metastases in both lobes (Figs. 40.6 and 40.7).

BIOPSY

- A liver ultrasound and biopsy were then performed to confirm liver metastases.
- The multiple fragments of core biopsy were read as positive for metastatic malignant melanoma.
- PET/CT confirmed no other sites suspicious for metastasis.

Updated Diagnosis: 17 months post–initial diagnosis of choroidal melanoma, multiple sites of liver metastasis were confirmed, despite definitive local control of the tumor via plaque brachytherapy.

A summary of the treatment of metastatic choroidal melanoma is provided in Table 40.2.

Treatment Options for Choroid Melanoma With Diffuse Liver Metastasis

- In general, drugs that are effective in cutaneous melanoma are less effective when used to treat choroid melanoma, but they can be considered.

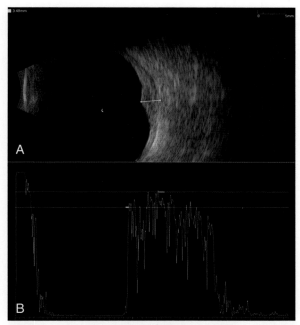

Fig. 40.5 Ultrasonography performed 2 years posttreatment with plaque brachytherapy. (A) Thickness of the lesion is measured at 3.48 mm compared to maximum thickness of 6.91 pretreatment. The scan of the lesion demonstrates high internal reflectivity. (B) The lesion is now solid.

- The optimal treatment approach for metastatic choroidal melanoma is evolving.
- When possible, enrollment in a clinical trial is recommended.
- Choice of therapy is a multidisciplinary decision based on a variety of factors: tumor location, rate of growth, tumor burden, HLA genotype assessment for HLA-A*02:01 (eligibility for tebentafusp), risk of toxicity and side effects, comorbid conditions, and alignment with the patient's goals for care.

SYSTEMIC TREATMENT

- Patient was offered nivolumab (6 mg/kg q 4 weeks) as systemic treatment for her metastatic disease.
- Locoregional treatment to the larger 2.5-cm mass with radiation was discussed but not offered given the multiple small, disseminated nodules in both liver lobes.
- Patient was very averse to potential toxicity and declined combination immunotherapy.

MANAGEMENT

- Side effects/toxicity: The patient developed fatigue, thyroiditis (hyperthyroid phase managed supportively, and hypothyroid phase managed with levothyroxine), and skin pruritus (managed with topical steroid cream) following cycle 1 of nivolumab. Hypophysitis developed 8 months into immunotherapy treatment, requiring prednisone for cortisol replacement.

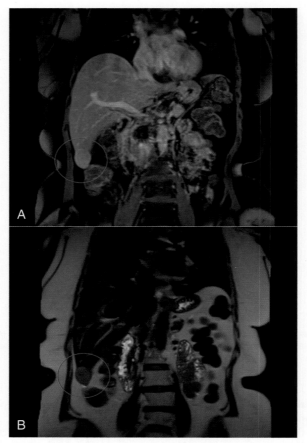

Fig. 40.6 (A) T1-weighted and (B) T2-weighted coronal MRI images depicting a hepatic metastasis in segment 6 of the inferior aspect of the liver.

- Tumor response: Follow-up PET/CT scan after 4 months of treatment showed a slight decrease in size of the main liver metastasis with stable multiple smaller hypermetabolic foci. Due to the documented response to treatment, the patient continued on nivolumab.
- Progression of disease: Follow-up PET/CT scan 2 years after initial diagnosis shows significant progression of disease with worsening of liver metastasis (Fig. 40.8).

NEXT STEPS

Given the immunotherapy toxicity and the interval progression of disease despite treatment, the decision was made to stop nivolumab. Discussion on additional treatment includes the following:

- Chemotherapy with carboplatin (Paraplatin)/paclitaxel (Taxol) is presented as an option but has no significant survival benefit.
- Restarting immunotherapy at a lower dose is also offered but is determined to not be a good option due to the patient's severe side effects and progression despite treatment.
- A requisition for HLA subtyping was completed to determine if the patient is a candidate for tebentafusp.
- Careful observation with repeat imaging is scheduled.

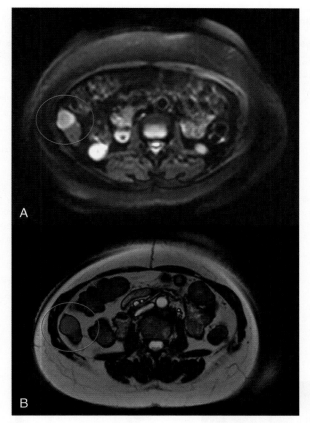

Fig. 40.7   (A) Axial diffusion weighted image (DWI) and corresponding (B) T2-weighted image showing inferior liver metastasis.

FOLLOW-UP

- Two months later, a PET/CT scan reveals significant progression, particularly in the liver with the dominant mass measuring over 10 cm and a moderately active lesion in the inter-trochanteric region of her left femur.
- The patient was offered options of chemotherapy with likely toxicity and lack of clinically meaningful benefit, rechallenge with immunotherapy, a trial of tebentafusp, or best supportive care.
- Due to the patient's Jehovah's Witness status and refusal to accept any blood products including albumin (co-administered), tebentafusp is not an option despite her HLA-A*02:01-positive status.

The patient decided to focus on optimization of symptom management as opposed to life-prolonging and cancer-directed therapies, and a referral to palliative care was made.

KEY POINTS

- The diagnosis of choroidal melanoma requires an accurate, comprehensive exam of the anterior and posterior segments in combination with multimodal imaging.

TABLE 40.2 ■ **Broad Categories of Treatment for Metastatic Choroidal Melanoma**

Category of Treatment	Description	Examples
ImmTAC (immune-mobilizing monoclonal T-cell receptor against cancer)	• Offered in patients with an HLA-A*02:01 genotype (testing required)	• Tebentafusp
Single-agent immunotherapy	• Patients may decline (due to increased toxicity risk) or be ineligible for combination immunotherapy • PD-1 or CTLA-4 inhibitors	• Nivolumab • Pembrolizumab • Ipilimumab
Combination immunotherapy	• Suggested that combination therapy results in better survival outcomes and response rates (limited evidence)	• Nivolumab + ipilimumab
Locoregional therapy for liver dominant disease	• Limited randomized trials exploring systemic therapies compared to locoregional therapies • Selection based on clinician and institutional practice patterns and expertise	• Embolization procedures • Ablative therapy (cryo or radiofrequency) • Radiation therapy • Surgical resection • HAI • IHP
Chemotherapy	• Rarely used due to poor response rates and no evidence to suggest improvement in overall survival	• Cisplatin • Dacarbazine

HAI, Hepatic arterial infusion of chemotherapy; *IHP,* isolated hepatic perfusion.

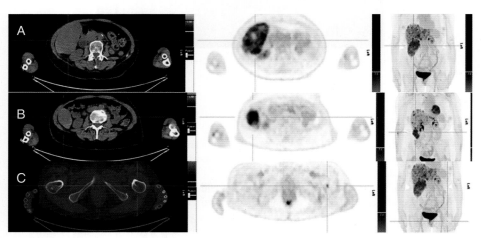

Fig. 40.8   PET/CT scan demonstrating hypermetabolic activity of (A, B) large liver metastasis with interval increase and (C) new area of hypermetabolic activity in the left femur likely representing bony metastasis.

■ Treatment of choroidal melanoma with either enucleation or plaque brachytherapy portends the same mortality risk, but careful discussion with the patient regarding diligent need for follow-up, the possibility of additional local treatment including transpupillary thermotherapy (TTT), and the regular administration of antivascular endothelial growth factor (anti-VEGF) intravitreal injections to address radiation retinopathy is essential.

- Molecular testing performed at the time of plaque brachytherapy can help guide systemic surveillance and discussions with patients regarding mortality and metastatic risk. In general, smaller lesions with class 1 gene expression profile or disomy 3 harbor the least metastatic risk, while larger lesions with class 2 GEPs or monosomy 3 lesions are associated with the highest risk.
- Treatment of choroidal melanoma with diffuse liver metastasis requires an interdisciplinary effort with locoregional and systemic therapies tailored to the patient's risk tolerance, goals of care, side-effect toxicity level, HLA status, and response to treatment.
- Prognosis is poor for patients with choroidal melanoma with diffuse metastasis, but long-term survival may improve with new advances in targeted therapy.

CHAPTER 41

Choroid Melanoma—Radiation Retinopathy

Amer F. Alsoudi ■ Henry C. Skrehot ■ Amy Schefler

New Cotton Wool Spots and Decreased Visual Acuity Post–Plaque Radiotherapy

HISTORY OF PRESENT ILLNESS

A 60-year-old male presents with decreased visual acuity in the right eye. His past medical history is significant for diabetes mellitus. His past ocular history was significant for a 9.5 mm r × 10.5 mm c × 1.6 mm h choroidal melanoma near the optic nerve treated with iodine-125 plaque radiotherapy 25 months prior to presentation. The patient has no other past ocular history.

Exam

	OD	OS
Visual acuity	20/80 PH: 20/40	20/20 PH: NI
IOP (mm Hg)	17	18
Sclera/conjunctiva	White and quiet	White and quiet
Cornea	Clear	Clear
AC	Normal depth and quiet	Normal depth and quiet
Iris	Within normal limits	Within normal limits
Lens	1+ NS	1+ NS
Anterior vitreous	Clear	Clear
Retina/optic nerve	Normal optic nerve, no holes or tears, no edema, treated choroidal melanoma abutting the optic nerve (2:00–4:00), scattered cotton wool spots, and intraretinal hemorrhages in the posterior pole	Normal optic nerve, posterior and peripheral retina

AC, Anterior chamber; *IOP,* intraocular pressure; *NI,* no improvement; *NS,* nuclear sclerosis; *PH,* pinhole.

QUESTIONS TO ASK

- What was the isotope/total radiation dose/fractionation schedule used for the treatment?
- Have you been diagnosed with any new illnesses (i.e., diabetes mellitus, hypertension, coronary artery disease)?
- What was your last HbA1c?

No authors have any financial interests related to the manuscript. No funding supports.

The patient has diabetes that is well controlled with metformin only, and the last HbA1c was 7.0%.

The patient was treated 25 months ago with an IsoAid (Port Richey, FL, United States) iodine-125 radioactive plaque. The tumor was treated to an apex height of 3.0 mm to achieve a coverage of 95.3% with a max scleral base dose of 175 Gy. The plaque was partially loaded with 24 seeds loaded and 5 anterior slots left unloaded. With this plan, the average dose to the macula was 30.4 Gy, and the average dose to the optic disc was 70.69 Gy.

ASSESSMENT

- Decreased visual acuity, OD
- New cotton wools spots, OD
- New intraretinal hemorrhages, OD

DIFFERENTIAL DIAGNOSIS

- Radiation retinopathy
- Diabetic retinopathy
- Hypertensive retinopathy
- Branch retinal vein occlusion
- Central retinal vein occlusion
- Neovascular age-related macular degeneration

WORKING DIAGNOSIS

- Radiation retinopathy, OD

INVESTIGATION, TESTING AND RESULTS

Before Antivascular Endothelial Growth Factor (Anti-VEGF) Treatment

- Fundus photo of the right eye depicting the fibrotic choroidal melanoma post–iodine-125 radiotherapy with new cotton wool spots and intraretinal hemorrhages. Fundus autofluorescence depicting a large well-circumscribed area of hypoautofluorescence representing the treated choroidal melanoma and scattered focal areas of hypoautofluorescence representing the new cotton wool spots (Fig. 41.1B).
- Spectral domain optical coherence tomography (SD-OCT) of the right eye depicting retinal thickening, atrophy, and central fovea involving intraretinal fluid (Fig. 41.2).
- B-scan ultrasound of the right eye depicting mild vitreous opacities, flat lesion at 3:00 posteriorly, 0.6-mm mass maximal height, no subretinal fluid over the lesion, no vascularity present, no extraocular extension (Fig. 41.3).
- Fluorescein angiography of the right eye depicting a large area of hyperfluorescence representing the treated choroidal mass (Fig. 41.4).
- Treatment setup and planned dose distribution of the target treated with iodine-125 radioactive plaque (Fig. 41.5).

After Antivascular Endothelial Growth Factor (Anti-VEGF) Treatment

- Fundus photo of the right eye depicting the treated choroidal melanoma abutting the optic nerve (2:00-4:00), with areas of surrounding fibrosis and patchy choroidal pigmentation (Fig. 41.5A–B). There is near resolution of the intraretinal hemorrhages and cotton-wool

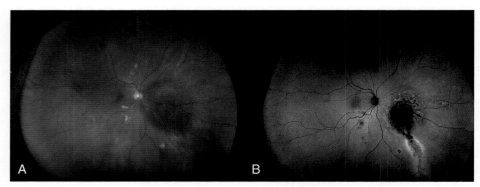

Fig. 41.1 Fundus photo (A) of the right eye depicting the fibrotic choroidal melanoma post iodine-125 radio-therapy with new cotton wool spots and intraretinal hemorrhages. Fundus autofluorescence (B) shows the circumscribed hypoautofluorescence of the treated melanoma and focal hypoautofluorescence from the cotton wool spots.

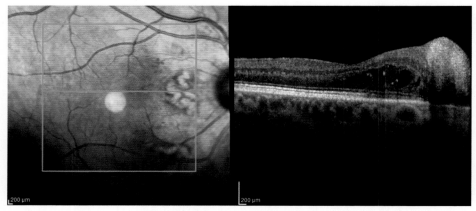

Fig. 41.2 Spectral domain optical coherence tomography (SD-OCT) of the right eye depicting retinal thickening, atrophy, and center-involving intraretinal fluid.

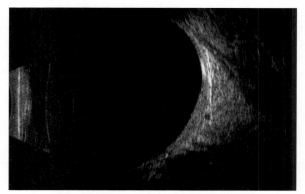

Fig. 41.3 B-scan ultrasound of the right eye depicting mild vitreous opacities, flat lesion at 3:00 posteriorly, 0.6-mm mass maximal height, no subretinal fluid over the lesion, no vascularity present, no extraocular extension.

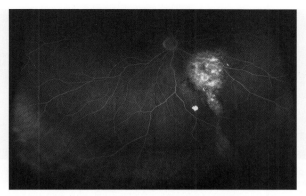

Fig. 41.4 Fluorescein angiography of the right eye depicting a large area of hyperfluorescence with gutter of previous fluid representing the treated choroidal mass.

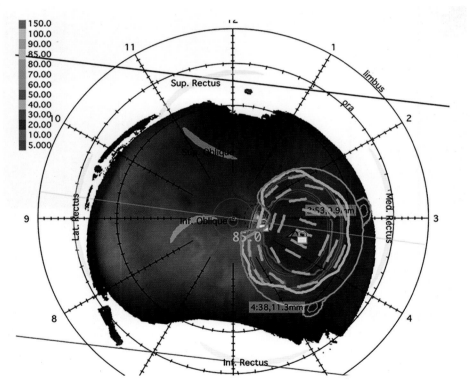

Fig. 41.5 Treatment setup and planned dose distribution of the target treated with iodine-125 radioactive plaque.

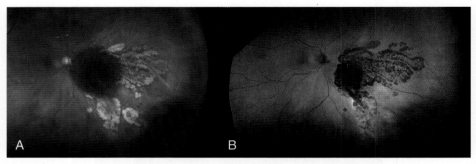

Fig. 41.6 Fundus photo of the right eye depicting treated choroidal melanoma abutting the optic nerve (2:00-4:00), with areas of surrounding fibrosis and patchy choroidal pigmentation. (A) There is near resolution of the intraretinal hemorrhages and cotton-wool spots. (B) Fundus autofluorescence depicting large well-circumscribed hypoautofluorescence representing the treated choroidal melanoma.

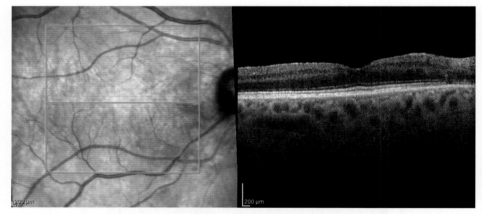

Fig. 41.7 Optical coherence tomography (OCT) of right eye macula depicting resolved intraretinal fluid.

spots (Fig. 41.6A). Fundus autofluorescence depicting large well-circumscribed hypoauto-fluorescence representing the treated choroidal melanoma (Fig. 41.6B).
- SD-OCT of the right eye depicting resolved intraretinal fluid (Fig. 41.7).

MANAGEMENT

- The patient was treated with intravitreal injection of bevacizumab (Avastin) 1.25 mg/0.05 mL in the right eye every 4 weeks for a total of six injections, with resolution of the intra-retinal fluid.

FOLLOW-UP

- More than 5 years after the initial presentation, the patient's right eye visual acuity was 20/25, and the left eye visual acuity was 20/20. The intraretinal hemorrhages and cotton wool spots have resolved. The intraretinal fluid has resolved.

KEY POINTS

■ Radiation retinopathy is a common and radiation dose–dependent complication of radiation therapy for ocular as well as head and neck cancers that generally develops between 6 months and 3 years posttreatment.

■ On clinical exam, radiation retinopathy may present with cotton wool spots, microaneurysms, telangiectasias, macular edema, optic disc edema, hard exudates, capillary nonperfusion, and retinal pigment epithelial atrophy.

■ Growing evidence suggests radiation retinopathy is best managed with anti-VEGF injections. However, there are no treatments approved by the US Food and Drug Administration, and there is still notable ambiguity in the standard of care for those patients affected by the disease.

■ Further work is required to understand optimal treatment regimens and the long-term durability of anti-VEGF injections for radiation retinopathy.

Retinoblastoma

CHAPTER 42

Retinoma

Ashwin Mallipatna ■ Mary Connolly-Wilson ■ Helen Dimaras

11-Year-Old Male With Retinal Mass

HISTORY OF PRESENT ILLNESS

Upon attending his first-ever routine eye examination, an 11-year-old male was found to harbor a white mass in his left eye. There was no history of ocular or systemic complaints.

Exam

	OD	OS
Visual acuity	20/20	20/20
IOP (mm Hg)	15	15
Sclera/conjunctiva	White and quiet	White and quiet
Cornea	Clear	Clear
AC	Deep and quiet	Deep and quiet
Iris	Unremarkable	Unremarkable
	Brown iris, pupil round	Brown iris, pupil round
Lens	Clear	Clear
Vitreous	Clear	3 vitreous seeds
Retina/optic nerve	Normal optic nerve, posterior and peripheral retina	Elevated, translucent gray retinal lesion with chorioretinal pigment disruption and calcification resembling cottage cheese

AC, Anterior chamber; *IOP,* intraocular pressure.

QUESTIONS TO ASK

- Is there a family history of retinoblastoma?
- Has anyone in the family had an ocular disease or cancer?
- Does the child have any symptoms?

There is no family history of retinoblastoma or other eye disease or cancer. The child is asymptomatic.

ASSESSMENT

- Elevated translucent gray retinal mass with calcification and surrounding atrophy
- No subretinal fluid

No financial interest associated with the manuscript. No funding supports.

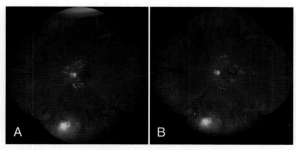

Fig. 42.1 (A) Fundus photographs taken at diagnosis, showing a white, translucent lesion with chorioretinal changes. (B) One year after diagnosis, fundus photographs showed no progression.

DIFFERENTIAL DIAGNOSIS

- Retinoblastoma
- Retinoma
- Astrocytoma
- Combined hamartoma of the retina and retinal pigment epithelium

WORKING DIAGNOSIS

- Retinoma

INVESTIGATION AND TESTING

Imaging

- Fundus photography (Fig. 42.1A)
- Optical coherence tomography (OCT) revealed the lesion had a height of 1.6 mm, was located within the retina, and had confirmed presence of calcification (Fig. 42.2A).
- Given the older age of the child, MRI of brain/orbit was deferred pending positive genetic testing results.

Genetic Testing (Blood)

- Blood was screened by high-sensitivity genetic assays to probe for the presence of a germ-line *RB1* pathogenic variant.

Screening of Parents and Siblings

- Dilated fundus exams of parents and siblings revealed normal retinae.

FOLLOW-UP

- The patient has been followed every 6 to 12 months with ophthalmoscopy and fundus photography (Fig. 42.1B) and optical coherence tomography (Fig. 42.2B).
  - The routine exams look for changes in size of the main lesion or seeds, vascularization, and retinal exudation.
  - At 18 months postdiagnosis, there has been no change noted in the lesion or seeds.
- The genetic test found no evidence of an any *RB1* pathogenic variant in the blood. Thus an MRI of head/orbits was not performed.

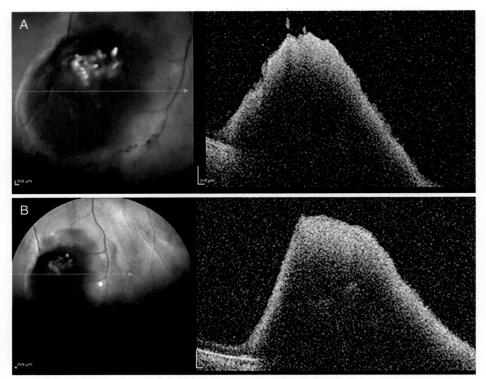

Fig. 42.2 (A) Optical coherence tomography at diagnosis, revealing intraretinal location of lesion and showing presence of seeding. (B) One year after diagnosis, optical coherence tomography shows no changes.

- The likelihood that a person affected with nonfamilial unilateral retinoma harbors a germline pathogenic variant of *RB1* is the same as someone with nonfamilial unilateral retinoblastoma—that is, 15%. The most sensitive genetic testing methods, such as those used to assess this patient, can identify an *RB1* pathogenic variant in blood for 96% of individuals believed to have a germline *RB1* pathogenic variant. Given that no pathogenic variant was identified, the likelihood that this patient harbors an undetectable germline pathogenic variant was reduced to less than 1%.

LIVED EXPERIENCE

The lived experience of disease is an important consideration for physicians in delivering high-quality care. The following points relate to the lived experience of retinoma, provided by an individual with a family history of retinoblastoma and an identified germline *RB1* pathogenic variant.

> *An individual with a retinoma is in an awkward place—not a cancer survivor but still potentially at risk for a second cancer if they harbor the RB1 pathogenic variant. Such an individual may have all the risks of those with known heritable retinoblastoma yet not recognized or considered as such by physicians who do not understand the situation. Physicians need to know about retinoblastoma and retinoma risks and advocate that their patients receive timely genetic testing and counseling.*

Key Points

CAUSE AND DEFINITION

- Initiated by biallelic loss of *RB1*, just as most retinoblastoma
- Is the benign precursor of retinoblastoma (not spontaneous regression of retinoblastoma, as initial reports described)
- Has clinically, histologically, and molecularly distinct features that distinguish it from retinoblastoma

POSSIBLE PRESENTATIONS OF RETINOMA

- In adults, it is often diagnosed because a child or other relative presents with retinoblastoma.
- In children, retinoma can be:
  - observed in fellow eye of retinoblastoma patient.
  - revealed following eye salvage treatment that causes the overlying malignant tumor to recede.
- Retinoma underlying retinoblastoma has been noted on histopathology, distinguished by its distinctive features (i.e., nonproliferative cells, presence of fleurettes).

RISK OF MALIGNANT TRANSFORMATION

- Progression of retinoma to retinoblastoma has been observed in a number of cases; thus frequent monitoring is recommended.
- Increasing thickness is predictive of malignant transformation of retinoma.

CHAPTER 43

Retinoblastoma—Unilateral Medium Grade

Gulunay Kiray ■ Mandeep Sagoo ■ Maddy Ashwin Reddy

Leukocoria With Exotropia in a 2-Year-Old Female Child

HISTORY OF PRESENT ILLNESS

A previously healthy 2-year-old female presents with left eye exotropia and leukocoria. Her parents noted the left eye turning out over the preceding year; however, they had decided to wait without reporting it to their family physician because the sister of the patient has had pseudostrabismus before. The patient's mother has recently noted an abnormal reflex in the left eye on some photos of the child. She has no prior ocular history or trauma to either eye.

She has been seen in a tertiary center as an outpatient and was referred to the retinoblastoma (Rb) center for an examination under anesthesia.

Exam

Orthoptics Examination		
	OD	**OS**
Visual acuity	0.1 with crowded LogMAR	1.3 with crowded LogMAR eccentric fixation
Prism cover test	Variable left exotropia	
Extraocular movements	Full in all directions	

Examination Under Anesthesia		
	OD	**OS**
IOP (mm Hg)	12	14
Horizontal corneal diameter (mm)	11	11
Sclera/conjunctiva	White and quiet	White and quiet
Cornea	Clear	Clear
AC	Deep and quiet	Deep and quiet
Iris	Pupil round and regular, no NVI	Pupil round and regular, no NVI
Lens	Clear	Clear
Retina/optic nerve	Normal optic disc, posterior pole and peripheral retina	Large white macular tumor at the posterior pole with subretinal and vitreous seeding (Fig. 43.1)

AC, Anterior chamber; IOP, intraocular pressure; NVI, neovascularization of the iris.

No financial interest associated with the manuscript. No funding supports.

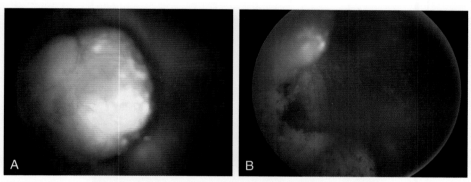

Fig. 43.1 (A) Large tumor at the posterior pole with vitreous seeding (spheres and dust). (B) Remaining retina showing retinal pigment epithelium (RPE) changes, RPE hyperplasia, and chorioretinal atrophy.

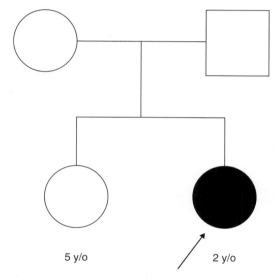

5 y/o   2 y/o

Fig. 43.2 Pedigree showing nonconsanguineous parents and unaffected older sister who is 5 years old.

QUESTIONS TO ASK

- Has your daughter ever had redness or pain in her left eye?
- Is there any history of blindness or enucleation in the family?
- Is there any history of cancer in the family?
- Does the child have any other relevant past medical history?
- Can you provide a detailed pedigree of the family? (Siblings will require screening until genetic data is available.)

The parents deny any pain or redness. There is no individual in the family who is blind or enucleated. There is no history of cancer in the family. Parents deny any other significant past medical history (Fig. 43.2).

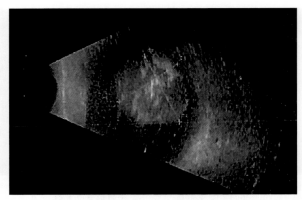

Fig. 43.3 B-scan ultrasound of the left eye showed a large intraocular mass with calcification that is covering two-thirds of the vitreous cavity, measuring 11.82 mm x 12.33 mm in base and 10.93 mm in height.

EXAMINATION OF PARENTS

Dilated fundoscopy of both parents was performed during the initial examination to rule out the following:
- Retinoma
- Inherited pseudoretinoblastoma conditions (e.g., familial exudative retinopathy [FEVR])

The examinations of the parents were unremarkable.

DIFFERENTIAL DIAGNOSIS

- Rb
- Medulloepithelioma
- Retinal astrocytic hamartoma
- Coats disease
- Persistent fetal vasculature (PFV)
- FEVR

WORKING DIAGNOSIS

- Rb—Group D cT2b

INVESTIGATION AND TESTING

- B-scan ultrasound of the left eye showed a large intraocular mass with calcification that is covering two-thirds of the vitreous cavity and measuring 11.82 mm x 12.33 mm in base and 10.93 mm in height (Fig. 43.3).
- MRI scan of the orbits and brain was used to rule out extraocular spread, including prelaminar invasion, and trilateral disease (pinealoblastoma).
- Genetic testing was used to exclude germline pathogenic variant of *RB1* gene.

MANAGEMENT

- The patient underwent three cycles of uneventful intraarterial chemotherapy (IAC) (melphalan 4 mg and topotecan 0.75 mg given in each cycle) in collaboration with the Departments of Pediatric Oncology and Interventional Radiology.

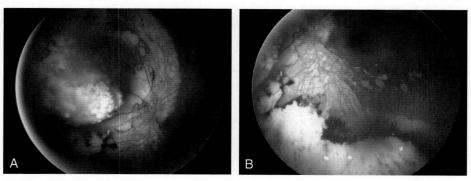

Fig. 43.4 (A) Regression of tumor after three cycles of intraarterial chemotherapy (IAC). Type 3 regression with calcification and fish flesh. (B) Calcified, inactive seeds inferiorly.

- Following IAC the main tumor had regressed (type 3 regression) and calcified. Seeds became calcified and inactive (Fig. 43.4).

FOLLOW-UP

- The patient did not require enucleation, meaning globe salvage has been achieved.
- No metastatic spread has been detected.
- Patient remained in remission at the age of 4.

KEY POINTS

- Rb is the most common primary intraocular malignancy of childhood, but it is an uncommon pediatric cancer, with a constant incidence worldwide of 1:15,000–1:20,000 live births.
- The majority of unilateral Rb cases are caused by sporadic loss-of-function pathogenic variants in both alleles of the RB transcriptional co-repressor 1 *(RB1)* gene in one precursor cone cell.
- However, 12–15% of unilateral cases do carry a germline *RB1* pathogenic variant. As a result, genetic testing is required for appropriate follow-up of patients and their siblings.
- The introduction of treatment modalities (e.g., IAC and intravitreal chemotherapy, the development of specialized centers, and the introduction of awareness campaigns) has resulted in nearly 100% survival in high-income countries and allowed eye salvage in many of the cases of Rb group D and less.

CHAPTER 44

Retinoblastoma—Unilateral High Grade

Bhavna Chawla ■ Kusumitha B. Ganesh

Protrusion of the Eye in a 3.5-Year-Old Female

HISTORY OF PRESENT ILLNESS

A 3.5-year-old female presented with complaints of pain, redness, and progressive protrusion of the left eye for about 1 month. Her parents gave a history of leukocoria in the left eye (Fig. 44.1), which was noticed over the past few weeks.

QUESTIONS TO ASK

- Does the child have any history of trauma to the eye?
- Has she shown any other symptoms suggestive of local or systemic infection?
- Is there any history of cancer in the family?
- Does the child have any other relevant past medical history?

The child had neither history of trauma nor any other symptoms suggestive of infection. She was the second-born child of a nonconsanguineous marriage with no history of cancer in any of the family members. Parents denied any other significant past medical history.

ASSESSMENT

- Proptosis, OS
- Severe scleral thinning with prominent episcleral vessels, OS
- Aqueous seedings with secondary glaucoma, OS

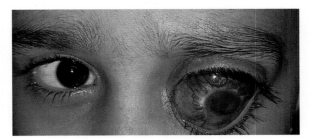

Fig. 44.1 Clinical photograph at presentation.

No financial interest associated with the manuscript. No funding supports.

Exam

	OD	OS
Visual acuity	Fixes and follows object	No perception of light
Eyeball	Normal in size and shape	Abaxial proptosis with restriction of extraocular movements (Fig. 44.1)
Conjunctiva	Normal	Congested
Cornea	Normal	Hazy cornea with hyphema in the anterior chamber

Exam Under Anesthesia

Anterior Segment Evaluation

	OD	OS
• Conjunctiva and sclera	Normal	Conjunctival congestion with prominent episcleral vessels and 360-degree scleral thinning
• Cornea	Normal in size and shape	Normal in size and shape
	Clear	Diffuse corneal edema
• AC	Deep and quiet	Diffuse hyphema with pseudohypopyon seen
• Iris	Unremarkable, pupil round, no NVI	Not visible
• IOP (mm Hg)	12	38
• Lens	Clear	Not visible

Posterior Segment Evaluation

	OD	OS
Fundus	Normal optic nerve, posterior and peripheral retina	Not visible

AC, Anterior chamber; *IOP,* intraocular pressure; *NVI,* neovascularization of the iris.

DIFFERENTIAL DIAGNOSIS

- Advanced retinoblastoma
- Orbital rhabdomyosarcoma
- Myeloid sarcoma/granulocytic sarcoma/chloroma
- Medulloepithelioma
- Endophthalmitis with neovascular glaucoma
- Advanced Coats' disease with neovascular glaucoma

INVESTIGATION AND TESTING

- B-scan ultrasonography showed a large intraocular mass with calcification in the posterior segment of the left eye (Fig. 44.2).
- MRI scans of the brain and orbit (contrast-enhanced, fat-suppressed images) showed a large, heterogeneous enhancing mass in the left globe with global expansion. The mass appeared to involve the ocular coats, with associated scleral breach. The left optic nerve showed thickening and enhancement up to the orbital apex (Fig. 44.3).
- Detailed general physical examination and systemic evaluation showed no systemic abnormality.
- Baseline blood investigations were normal.
- Chest x-ray, ultrasonography of the abdomen, bone marrow biopsy, and cerebrospinal fluid cytology ruled out any hematogenous/central nervous system (CNS) metastasis.

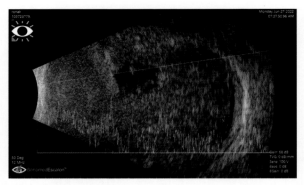

Fig. 44.2 Ultrasonography of the left globe showing a large intraocular mass in the posterior segment, with high-amplitude spikes suggestive of calcification.

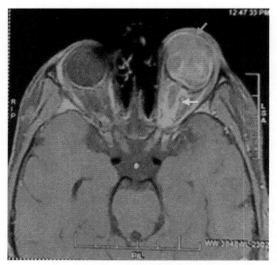

Fig. 44.3 Axial magnetic resonance imaging scan of the orbits and brain showing a large, heterogenous enhancing mass in the left eye with global expansion *(blue arrow)*. The mass appeared to involve the ocular coats, with presence of scleral breach. The left optic nerve showed thickening and enhancement up to the orbital apex *(yellow arrow)*.

DIAGNOSIS

International Retinoblastoma Staging System (IRSS) stage IIIA extraocular retinoblastoma OS

MANAGEMENT

The steps are outlined in Fig. 44.4.

- The patient was advised neoadjuvant intravenous chemotherapy cycles consisting of three drugs: vincristine 0.025 mg/kg on day 1, carboplatin 28 mg/kg on day 1, etoposide 12 mg/kg on days 1 and 2, administered every 4 weeks.

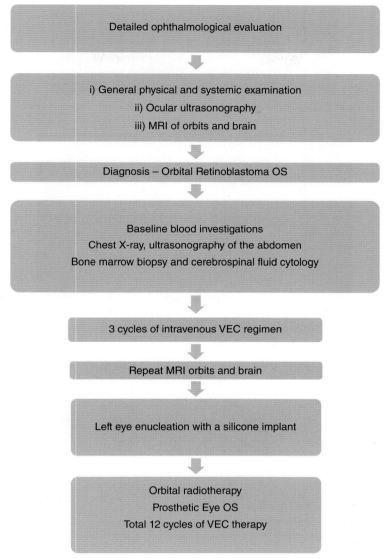

Fig. 44.4 Flow chart showing the steps of management. *VEC,* vincristine, etoposide, carboplatin.

- After three cycles of intravenous chemotherapy, the mass showed a significant reduction (Fig. 44.5). A repeat MRI scan of the orbit confirmed a small shrunken globe and optic nerve thickening that was now reduced to the proximal part of the optic nerve (Fig. 44.6).
- The patient underwent enucleation surgery of the left phthisical globe, and a silicone implant was placed. Histopathology of the enucleated specimen revealed a poorly differentiated retinoblastoma (Fig. 44.7) showing extensive necrosis and calcification. The optic nerve, including its resected margin, was free of tumor.

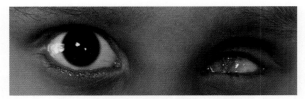

Fig. 44.5 Clinical photograph after three cycles of intravenous chemotherapy.

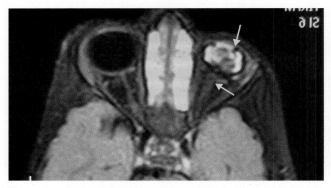

Fig. 44.6 Axial MRI scan showing a small shrunken globe on the left side *(arrow)* with optic nerve thickening reduced to the proximal part *(arrow)*.

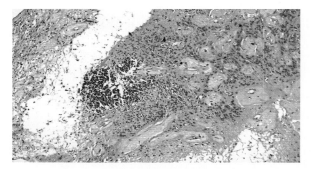

Fig. 44.7 Histopathology section (H&E) of the left enucleated eye reveals poorly differentiated retinoblastoma cells *(red arrow)* with surrounding extensive necrosis. Courtesy of Dr. Seema Sen, AIIMS.

- The patient received orbital external beam radiotherapy (40 cGY in divided fractions) within 30 days of the surgery. A prosthetic eye was fitted in the left socket at 6 weeks post-surgery.
- Thereafter, intravenous chemotherapy with vincristine, etoposide, carboplatin (VEC) drugs was continued for a total of 12 cycles.

FOLLOW-UP

- The patient did not require any further treatment and has remained stable on follow-up. There is no evidence of local recurrence or hematogenous or CNS metastasis. The right eye is normal.

KEY POINTS

- Extraocular retinoblastoma is quite common in the developing world. These children usually present at a later age (30–38 months), as compared to intraocular retinoblastoma.
- Proptosis, pain, redness, swelling of the eye, and leukocoria are the most common presenting symptoms of orbital retinoblastoma.
- Ophthalmological evaluation, ultrasonography of the eye, and MRI of the orbit and brain help confirm the diagnosis and determine its extent.
- A thorough physical examination, palpation of regional lymph nodes, and investigations such as chest x-ray, ultrasound of the abdomen, blood biochemistry, bone marrow biopsy, and cerebrospinal fluid cytology are recommended to stage the disease.
- Technetium-99 bone scan and positron emission tomography (PET) coupled with computed tomography (CT) may be useful for the early detection of subclinical systemic metastasis.
- In the past, orbital retinoblastoma carried a poor prognosis with high mortality rates.
- A multimodal approach that involves a sequential combination of intravenous chemotherapy, enucleation surgery, external beam radiotherapy to the affected orbit, and adjuvant systemic chemotherapy has improved survival outcomes in children with extraocular retinoblastoma.
- Long-term follow-up is recommended in children with extraocular retinoblastoma for early detection of local recurrence and systemic metastasis.

CHAPTER 45

Retinoblastoma—Unilateral With High-Risk Features

Linda A. Cernichiaro-Espinosa ■ Hart G.W. Lidov ■ Junne Kamihara
■ Efren Gonzalez

Right Eye Leukocoria in a 4-Year-Old Child

HISTORY OF PRESENT ILLNESS

A 4-year-old male was found to have OD leukocoria after a referral to ophthalmology for a failed visual exam. His family had noted that his pupil had seemed more opaque notably over the last 2 months. A dilated office exam demonstrated concern for retinoblastoma (RB) with elevated intraocular pressure (IOP; OD: 33 mm Hg and OS 16 mm Hg). Further workup was planned. He presented 3 days later to the emergency room with worsening eye pain, new periorbital swelling, and increased sleepiness. Steroids were initiated. Exam under anesthesia (EUA) was performed the following day (Fig. 45.1).

Exam Under Anesthesia

	OD	OS
IOP (mm Hg)	17 mm Hg	12 mm Hg
Sclera/conjunctiva	Chemosis, conjunctival hyperemia and ciliary injection	Clear
Cornea	Opaque cornea that allowed partial visualization of the AC	Clear
AC	Dispersed anterior chamber cellularity in the supine position	Normal
Iris	Rubeosis iridis, mid-dilated pupil	Normal
Lens	Clear	Clear
Anterior vitreous	Yellow-to-white vascularized retinal lesion touching the lens	Normal
Retina/optic nerve		Normal

AC, Anterior chamber; IOP, intraocular pressure.

QUESTIONS TO ASK

- Did the child experience any trauma to the eye?
- Was there any eye pain, fever, or other symptoms?
- Is there a history of blindness or other visual problems in childhood in the family?

The child did not experience any trauma. Prior to current presentation, there was no fever or ocular pain. There was no family history of ocular disease.

No financial interest associated with the manuscript. No funding supports.

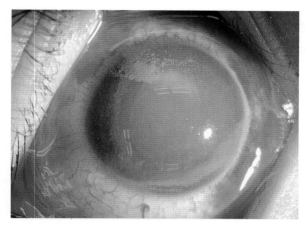

Fig. 45.1 Ophthalmic exam under anesthesia (EUA).

ASSESSMENT

- Orbital cellulitis, OD
- Glaucoma, OD
- Panuveitis, OD
- Retinal lesion, OD

DIFFERENTIAL DIAGNOSIS

See Table 45.1.

TABLE 45.1 ■ **Clinical Differential Diagnosis**

Clinical Differential Diagnosis	Etiology	Rationale
Orbital cellulitis	~~Infectious~~	Lack of fever or conjunctival secretion.
	~~Inflammatory~~	Primary inflammation felt to be unlikely due to intraocular findings.
	Neoplastic	The inflammation was felt to be due to rapid growth accompanying necrosis of an RB tumor causing an aseptic orbital cellulitis.
Glaucoma	~~Congenital~~	No buphthalmic eye, no Haab striae, absence of photophobia and intraocular findings that rule it out (seeds, posterior pole lesion).
	Secondary neovascular glaucoma	The inflammation and the AC seeding, along with the anterior displacement of the lens-iris diaphragm could cause a closed-angle glaucoma. Rubeosis iridis denotes chronicity. Ocular ischemic events can result in rubeosis iridis or neovascular glaucoma (i.e., Coats disease, chronic retinal detachment, or chronic uveitis). Rubeosis iridis and/or neovascular glaucoma in young infants should raise suspicion for intraocular neoplasia.
Panuveitis	~~Infectious~~	Anterior cellularity in infective uveitis typically causes a hypopyon that does not shift with head position.
	~~Inflammatory~~	No keratic precipitates, absence of synechiae, atypical cells from seeds causing pseudohypopion and posterior pole lesion highly suggestive of a tumor. Pseudohypopion is an accumulation of neoplastic cellularity that shifts with head position.
	Neoplastic	The anterior cellularity is from dust and sphere RB seeds causing a pseudohypopion.

Continued

TABLE 45.1 ■ cont'd

Clinical Differential Diagnosis	Etiology	Rationale
Retinal lesion	~~Retinal detachment~~	In children, a retinal detachment is usually due to trauma or a congenital cause (i.e., familial exudative vitreoretinopathy). In the absence of trauma, family history, high myopia, and other causes of retinal detachments, RB must be ruled out. The B-scan would identify an associated solid lesion, if present.
	~~Coats disease~~	Coats disease causes a spectrum of unilateral exudative retinal detachment with retinal malformations. Fluorescein angiography is usually diagnostic by displaying filling hyperfluorescence from the vascular abnormalities. The anterior chamber seeds and the absence of vascular malformations make Coats disease unlikely.
	Neoplastic	The presence of complete retinal detachment, a vascularized mass touching the posterior lens, and the AC findings are all consistent with RB.

AC, Anterior chamber; *RB,* retinoblastoma.

WORKING DIAGNOSIS

Group E Retinoblastoma OD (AJCC cT3e aseptic orbital cellulitis)

INVESTIGATION AND TESTING

See Table 45.2.

TABLE 45.2 ■ Tests and Results

Test	Result	
MRI	Right hyperintense T1-weighted and hypointense T2-weighted solid mass that enhanced after gadolinium (Fig. 45.2)	
EUA	Ophthalmic exam	Performed the day after the office exam, as above, depicted an IOP of 17 mm Hg post–steroid initiation with dispersed AC seeds (Fig. 45.1).
	UBM	Seeds in the anterior chamber and tumor invasion of the zonula with a mild lens displacement, without evidence of ciliary body invasion (Fig. 45.3)
	B-scan ultrasound	A solid mass occupying the entire volume of the vitreous cavity with hyperechogenic lesions suggestive of intralesional calcium (Fig. 45.4)

AC, Anterior chamber; *IOP,* intraocular pressure; *UBM,* ultrabiomicroscopy.

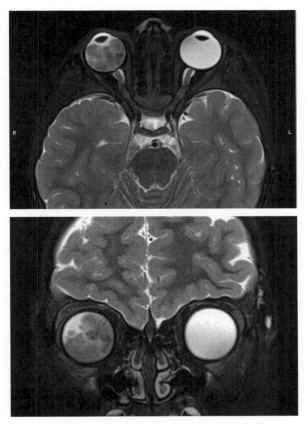

Fig. 45.2 (A) T2-weighted axial and (B) coronal MRI.

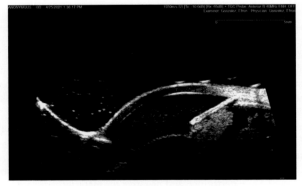

Fig. 45.3 Ultrabiomicroscopy (UBM).

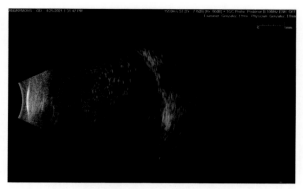

Fig. 45.4 B-scan ultrasound.

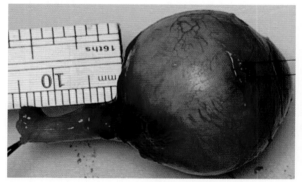

Fig. 45.5 Enucleated OD with 15.5-mm optic nerve stump without macroscopic evidence of extraocular disease.

MANAGEMENT

- After discussion with the family, primary enucleation of the right eye was performed with an optic nerve stump of 15.5 mm (Fig. 45.5). There were no complications. A silicone orbital implant was placed.
- Histopathology with hematoxylin and eosin (H&E) and periodic acid-Schiff (PAS) staining demonstrated a mostly endophytic RB replacing normal retina with extensive necrosis, and optic nerve involvement posterior to the lamina cribrosa (PLONI), a high-risk histopathologic feature, with no meningeal invasion (Figs. 45.6 and 45.7).
- Germline testing confirmed the absence of an *RB1* pathogenic variant. Tumor testing demonstrated a splice site variant and a nonsense variant, both felt likely to represent loss of function alterations.
- Further staging studies including lumbar puncture, bilateral bone marrow aspirates/biopsies, and bone scan were performed and negative for metastatic disease.
- Final clinical staging: AJCC cT3e cN0 cM0 H0 pT3a.
- The patient received six cycles of vincristine, etoposide, and carboplatin dosed per the Children's Oncology Group (COG) protocol ARET0332 (vincristine 1.5 mg/m², etoposide 150 mg/m², and carboplatin 560 mg/m²) every 28 days (Chevaz-Barrios et al., 2019).

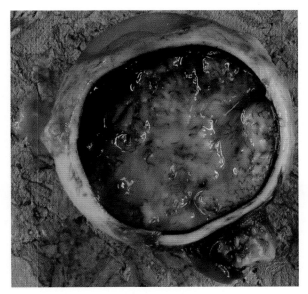

Fig. 45.6   Gross appearance of the enucleated eye.

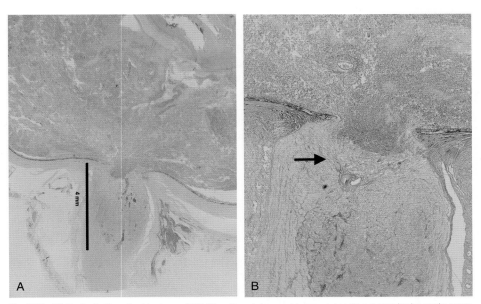

Fig. 45.7   (A) Endophytic retinoblastoma (RB) filling the globe, and tumor extending 4 mm in the optic nerve involvement posterior to the lamina cribrosa (PLONI), H&E staining 1.25x. (B) Higher magnification of lamina cribrosa *(arrow)* breached by tumor, periodic acid-Schiff (PAS) 4x.

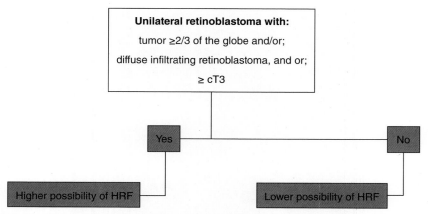

Fig. 45.8 Possibility of having high-risk histopathological features in an eye with advanced intraocular retino-blastoma (RB). Based on Tomar et al. (2022).

FOLLOW-UP

- The patient tolerated the chemotherapy well without any dose-limiting toxicity. He has been followed closely for over 2 years without recurrence. He has a well-fitted ocular prosthesis.

ALGORITHMS

- Tomar et al. (2022) reported that AJCC clinical RB stage of cT3c or higher, tumor more than two-thirds of globe volume, and diffuse infiltrative RB could be utilized to predict the possibility of having high-risk histopathological features (pT3 or higher) (Fig. 45.8). Up-front enucleation allows for unambiguous determination of the presence of high-risk pathologic features, although eye salvage regimens are also being pursued. Randomized prospective data are needed to address the safety, morbidity, and long-term outcomes of up-front enucleation versus eye salvage, as well as to further optimize risk-stratification therapies when high-risk features are identified.

KEY POINTS

- A proper diagnosis of RB is mandatory to decrease delay in treatment.
- The presence of high-risk histopathologic features has been associated with the risk of developing metastatic disease. Metastatic retinoblastoma that has spread beyond the globe has higher mortality rates and more intensive regimens are needed for treatment (Dunkel et al., 2022).
- A tumor occupying more than two-thirds of the globe, diffuse infiltrating RB, and clinical tumor grading of ≥cT3c (raised IOP with neovascularization and/or buphthalmos) are clinical features of advanced intraocular RB that have been demonstrated to correlate with the presence of high-risk histopathological features (pT3 or higher) (Tomar et al., 2022).
- The presence of tumor cells in the optic nerve posterior to the lamina cribosa (PLONI) is widely accepted to be a high-risk histopathologic feature, and most centers give adjuvant chemotherapy in this setting to reduce the risk of metastatic recurrence (Kaiki et al., 2022; Dittner-Moormann et al., 2021).

- Other high-risk factors include tumor cells in orbital tissues and at the cut end of the optic nerve. Additional findings that have been proposed in isolation or in combination include scleral, uveal tract, and anterior segment involvement. Efforts are underway to harmonize definitions and define the levels of risk correlating with the presence of these histopathologic findings (Chévez-Barrios et al., 2019).
- Genetic testing in all patients with RB, including patients with unilateral disease, offers more precise guidance on the frequency of ophthalmological exams under anesthesia, and further surveillance is needed.
- Multidisicplinary care with pediatric oncology allows for staging, risk-adapted therapy, and long-term follow-up care after treatment.

Suggested Reading

Kaliki S, Shields CL, Cassoux N, et al. Defining High-risk Retinoblastoma: A Multicenter Global Survey. *JAMA Ophthalmol*, 2022;140(1):30–36.

Dittner-Moormann S, Reschke M, Abbink FCH, et al. Adjuvant therapy of histopatological risk factors of retinobasotoma in Europe: A survey by the European Retinoblastoma Group (EURbG). *Pediatr Blood Cancer*, 2021; 68(6), e28963.

Dunkel IJ, Piao J, Chantada GL, et al. Intensive Multimodality Therapy for Extraocular Retinoblastoma: A Children's Oncology Group Trial (ARET0321). *J Clin Oncol*, 2022;40(33):3839–3847.

Chévez-Barrios P, Eagle RC Jr, Krailo M, et al. Study of unilateral retinoblastoma with and without histopathologic high-risk features and the role of adjuvant chemotherapy: A children's oncology group study. *J Clin Oncol*. 2019;37(31):2883–2891. doi:10.1200/JCO.18.01808. Epub 2019 Sep 20. PMID: 31539297; PMCID: PMC6823888.

Tomar AS, Finger PT, Gallie B, et al. High-risk pathologic features based on presenting findings in Advanced intraocular retinoblastoma: A multicenter, international data-sharing American Joint Committee on Cancer study. *Ophthalmology*. 2022 Aug;129(8):923–932. doi:10.1016/j.ophtha.2022.04.006. Epub 2022 Apr 15. PMID: 35436535; PMCID: PMC9329269.

CHAPTER 46

Retinoblastoma—Vitreous Seeding

Sarah Beth Pike ■ Christopher Patrick Long ■ Jesse L. Berry

Unilateral Leukocoria in a 17-Month-Old Female

HISTORY OF PRESENT ILLNESS

A previously healthy 17-month-old female presented with leukocoria OD. Patient's parents first noticed the leukocoria OD about 2 weeks prior. The patient was initially seen by an outside provider who referred her for further evaluation.

Exam

Anterior Exam[a]		
	OD	**OS**
IOP (mm Hg)	15	14
Lid/lashes	Normal	Normal
Sclera/conjunctiva	White and quiet	White and quiet
Cornea	Clear	Clear
AC	Formed, no hypopyon	Formed, no hypopyon
Iris	No obvious neovascularization	No obvious neovascularization
Lens	Clear	Clear
Dilated Fundus Exam[a]		
	OD	**OS**
Optic nerve	View obscured by retinal mass	Sharp and pink
Retina[b]	Large, creamy, white endophytic lesion with intralesional vasculature filling vitreous cavity and blocking view of other normal structures (Fig. 46.1A)	Flat macula; no evidence of mass or other abnormalities (Fig. 46.1B)
Vitreous	Seeding in all four quadrants, primarily dust morphology (Fig. 46.1C)	Normal

AC, Anterior chamber; IOP, intraocular pressure.
[a]Performed under anesthesia.
[b]360 scleral depressed exam.

No financial interests associated with the manuscript.

Dr. Berry has grant support not directly related to the scope of this report from the National Cancer Institute of the National Institute of Health Award Number K08CA232344, The Wright Foundation, Children's Oncology Group/St. Baldrick's Foundation, The Knights Templar Eye Foundation, Hyundai Hope on Wheels, Childhood Eye Cancer Trust, and Children's Cancer Research Fund. Dr. Berry has other research support from The Berle & Lucy Adams Chair in Cancer Research, The Larry and Celia Moh Foundation, The Institute for Families, Inc., Children's Hospital Los Angeles, an unrestricted departmental grant from Research to Prevent Blindness, and The National Cancer Institute P30CA014089. Dr. Berry has filed a provisional patent application entitled Aqueous Humor Cell Free DNA for Diagnostic and Prognostic Evaluation of Ophthalmic Disease 62/654,160 (Berry, Xu, Hicks).

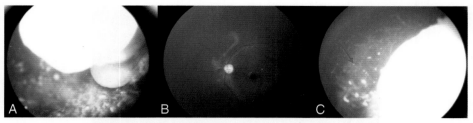

Fig. 46.1 Diagnostic fundus images taken during examination under anesthesia of the right and left eyes at the time of diagnosis. (A) The large, white, endophytic, retinal-based tumor in the right eye, which extends anteriorly and abuts the lens. (B) The normal left posterior pole. (C) Diffuse seeding with a dust morphology can be seen in the right eye *(red arrow)*.

QUESTIONS TO ASK

- How long have you noted the white reflex?
- Have you ever noticed any redness or inflammation of the right eye?
- Have you ever noticed that the eyes are crossed or one of the eyes is drifting out?
- Is there any family history of ocular diseases or cancers?
- Has there been any recent trauma?
- Has there been any history of weight loss, vomiting, or seizures?
- Are there any siblings?

The patient's parents have never noticed any redness or inflammation OD or any changes OS. They think that the eyes have been aligned. The patient has no family history of ocular diseases or cancers. The patient has no significant medical history.

ASSESSMENT

- Large, retinal-based, calcified mass filling the globe OD with diffuse seeding

DIFFERENTIAL DIAGNOSIS

- Retinoblastoma
- Medulloepithelioma
- Astrocytic hamartoma
- Coats disease
- Ocular toxocariasis
- Persistent fetal vasculature

WORKING DIAGNOSIS

- Advanced International Intraocular Retinoblastoma Classification (IIRC) Group D retinoblastoma (RB) with dust-shaped vitreous seeding, OD

INVESTIGATION AND TESTING

- Examination under anesthesia (EUA) for evaluation and staging was done.
- There was no buphthalmos, the corneas measured 11 mm × 11 mm OU, and pressure was 15 OD and 14 OS.
- B-scan ultrasound OD showed a 13.1 mm × 18.03 mm dome-shaped, retinal-based tumor with diffuse intralesional calcification (Fig. 46.2).

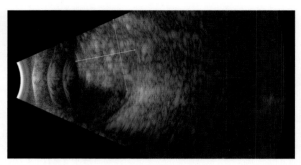

Fig. 46.2 Diagnostic B-scan ultrasound image of the right eye taken during examination under anesthesia. A retinal-based dome-shaped mass is visible, measuring 13.1 mm × 18.03 mm. Intralesional calcification can be seen scattered throughout the mass.

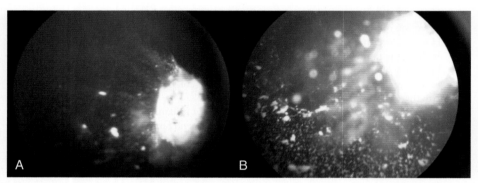

Fig. 46.3 Series of two fundus images taken at examinations under anesthesia during the patient's first set of intravitreal melphalan chemotherapy (IVM) injections for refractory seeding in the right eye. (A) Demonstrates seeding, primarily of dust morphology, noted 4 months after diagnosis; the image was taken at the time of IVM injection number one. Calcified vitreous seeding can be seen in all four quadrants with a consolidated area of vitreous haze noted inferiorly to the main tumor. (B) The seeding appears regressed from the prior exams after a series of three IVM injections spaced 4 weeks apart.

- Ultrasound biomicroscopy showed the tumor extending forward close to the lens, but not anteriorly to the anterior vitreous face, without ciliary body involvement.
- Fluorescein angiography revealed subclinical neovascularization of the iris in the prepapillary area OD with diffuse leakage over the tumor mass. Pressure, however, was normal.
- MRI of brain and orbits with and without contrast revealed a heterogeneously enhancing mass in the right globe, consistent with RB, without evidence of optic nerve involvement or extraocular spread of disease.
- Serum genetic testing revealed a pathogenic germline *RB1* mutation.

MANAGEMENT

- Systemic intravenous (IV) chemotherapy with a combination of vincristine, etoposide, and carboplatin (VEC) was begun and continued for six cycles, each spaced 4 weeks apart.
- Patient was monitored with EUAs at 4-week intervals during chemotherapy, and focal laser consolidation therapy was used for chemoreduction as needed.
- Refractory seeding was noted on exam during systemic IV chemotherapy cycle number four, 4 months after diagnosis (Fig. 46.3A). Thus intravitreal injection of chemotherapy

TABLE 46.1 ■ **Longitudinal Aqueous Humor Tumor Fraction Analysis of All Samples Collected From the Right Eye During Injections With Intravitreal Melphalan Chemotherapy**

Intravitreal Melphalan (IVM) Injection Number	Tumor Fraction
IVM 1	0.33
IVM 2	0.22
IVM 3	0.07
IVM 4	0.10[a]
IVM 5	0.09
IVM 6	0.03

[a]There was a relative increase in tumor fraction between aqueous humor taken at IVM 3, when seeding was noted to be regressed with IVM therapy, and IVM 4, when active seeding was again noted on exam. Overall, there was a downtrend in tumor fraction values throughout IVM treatment, indicating a positive response.

with 25 µg of melphalan was started and planned for a total of three sessions, alongside IV chemotherapy cycles 4, 5, and 6.

■ At the time of each intravitreal melphalan (IVM) injection, 0.1 cc of aqueous humor (AH) was collected from the anterior chamber OD via clear corneal paracentesis.

■ AH was analyzed by shallow whole genome sequencing to look for highly recurrent RB-associated somatic copy number alterations (SCNAs) used to determine tumor fraction, a measurement that can be trended longitudinally to monitor treatment response.[1,2] The patient was positive for three known RB SCNAs: gain-of-copy of chromosomes 1q, 2p, and 6p.

■ After three injections of IVM were completed, the seeds OD appeared calcified and vitreous haze was stable (Fig. 46.3B).

■ AH collected at each of the three IVM injections was analyzed for tumor fraction with a continuous downtrend in values (Table 46.1), suggestive of decreased tumor activity and treatment response.

FOLLOW-UP

■ The eye was monitored for 3 months and treated with laser for focal consolidation, until an increase in seeding at the center of the vitreous was noted on exam (Fig. 46.4).

■ IVM injections were resumed for an additional three cycles spaced 4 weeks apart.

■ Analysis of AH collected at the fourth injection of IVM showed an increase in tumor fraction relative to AH collected at the third injection of IVM (Table 46.1), reflecting the interim increase in tumor seeding.

■ Vitreous debris decreased at each subsequent exam throughout IVM injections four, five, and six, and tumor fraction also continued to decline, suggesting response to treatment (Table 46.1).

■ The exam 12 months after diagnosis and 1 month after the sixth IVM injection showed no evidence of active seeds or retinal foci (Fig. 46.5).

■ At the most recent follow-up, 4 years after diagnosis and 3 years after the completion of IVM injection six, patient had no evidence of disease activity on exam, B-scan ultrasound, or optical coherence tomography (OCT). Although the patient has a germline *RB1* mutation, which predisposes her to an increased risk of bilateral disease development, there continues to be no evidence of cancer in the healthy left eye.

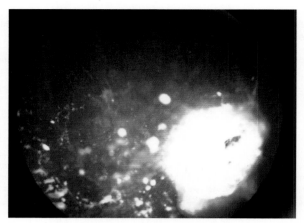

Fig. 46.4 Fundus photo demonstrating increased vitreous seeding in the right eye, which was noted after 3 months of observation. Thus, an additional three injections of intravitreal chemotherapy with melphalan (IVM) were initiated.

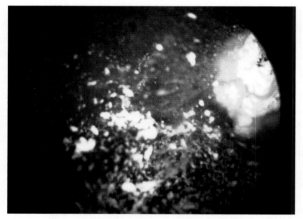

Fig. 46.5 Fundus photo of the stable right eye taken 12 months after initial diagnosis. In the image, the calcified and regressed endophytic lesion arising from the superonasal fundus is visible. Significant calcified vitreous seeding can be seen in all four quadrants. There is no evidence of active tumor seeding or retinal foci.

KEY POINTS

- Any child with leukocoria should be evaluated urgently with dilated fundus examination.
- The presence of seeding in RB suggests more advanced disease. Seeding is difficult to treat because tumor seeds float free in the vitreous without a blood supply, so they are not directly exposed to systemic or intraarterial chemotherapy. Seeds are considered the primary reason for treatment failure and need for enucleation.
- Seeds come in multiple morphologies. Listed from least to most difficult to treat, these morphologies include dust, sphere, and cloud.
- RB with seeding can be treated first with intravenous chemotherapy or intraarterial chemotherapy, followed by intravitreal injection of chemotherapy for refractory seeding.

- Intravitreal melphalan toxicity mainly occurs at doses greater than 30 μg; side effects include retinopathy, subretinal/vitreous hemorrhage, and, rarely, hypotonia or phthisis. Doses of 20–30 μg are generally well tolerated.
- Direct tumor biopsy in RB is contraindicated to prevent extraocular tumor spread, but AH is established as a liquid biopsy source of tumor information that can be assayed in the absence of tissue. Prognostic biomarkers for RB have been established using cell-free DNA in AH, including the use of SCNAs to determine tumor fraction, which is highly predictive of disease progression if a relative 15% increase from baseline seen.[1] A decrease in tumor fraction suggests positive treatment response and disease regression, as seen in this case.[2]

References

1. Berry JL, Xu L, Murphree AL, et al. Potential of aqueous humor as a surrogate tumor biopsy for retino-blastoma. *JAMA Ophthalmol.* 2017;135(11):1221–1230. doi:10.1001/jamaophthalmol.2017.4097.
2. Polski A, Xu L, Prabakar RK, et al. Cell-Free DNA tumor fraction in the aqueous humor is associated with therapeutic response in retinoblastoma patients. *Transl Vis Sci Technol.* 2020;9(10):30. doi:10.1167/tvst.9.10.30.

CHAPTER 47

Retinoblastoma—Bilateral Medium Grade

Mattan Arazi ■ Ido Didi Fabian

Strabismus in a 9-Month-Old Infant

HISTORY OF PRESENT ILLNESS

A previously healthy 9-month-old White male infant presents with strabismus first noticed by his parents 4 weeks ago. The infant was born at term by an uncomplicated C-section. He had no prior systemic or ocular history and was fully vaccinated to his age.

Exam

	OD	OS
Visual acuity	No Fix-and-Follow	No Fix-and-Follow
IOP (mm Hg) under anesthesia	8	9
Conjunctiva	Quiet	Quiet
Cornea	Clear	Clear
AC	Deep and quiet	Deep and quiet
Iris	Normal, no NVI	Normal, no NVI
Lens	Clear	Clear
Pupil	Round and reactive	Round and reactive
Vitreous	Clear	Clear
Fundus	White mass with large retinal detachment and suspected subretinal seeds. Optic disc not visible (Fig. 47.1A)	White mass with large retinal detachment and suspected subretinal seeds. Optic disc not visible (Fig. 47.1B)

AC, Anterior chamber; *IOP*, intraocular pressure; *NVI*, neovascularization of the iris.

QUESTIONS TO ASK

- Is there any relevant family history of retinoblastoma?
- Is there any history of other ocular disorders in the family?
- Is there any history of trauma?

There was no history of retinoblastoma in the family and no history of other ocular disorders or trauma.

No financial interest associated with the manuscript. No funding supports.

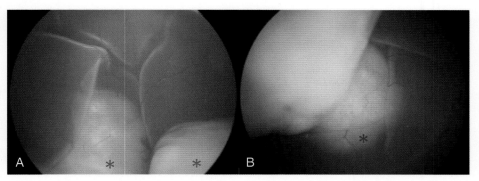

Fig. 47.1 (A) Right eye demonstrating two cream-colored exophytic vascularized masses *(red asterisks)*, with main tumor temporally located extending into fovea. (B) Left eye showing a nasally located vascularized exophytic white mass *(blue asterisk)*, with subretinal fluid extending into the fovea *(not shown)*.

ASSESSMENT

- White mass(es) with full retinal detachment and suspected subretinal seeds, OU

DIFFERENTIAL DIAGNOSIS

- Bilateral retinoblastoma
- Bilateral Coats disease
- Bilateral vitreous hemorrhage
- Bilateral retinal detachment
- Retinopathy of prematurity

WORKING DIAGNOSIS

- Bilateral retinoblastoma

INVESTIGATION AND TESTING

- B-scan ultrasonography OU demonstrated echogenic retinal masses with highly reflective foci (OD main mass 13.1 mm × 9.0 mm, OS 9.7 mm × 16.4 mm) adjacent to detached retina. MR scan ruled out a suspicious intracranial primitive neuroectodermal tumor and showed no extraocular extension of the tumors.
- Lumbar puncture showed no retinoblastoma cells in the cerebrospinal fluid (CSF).
- Genetic tests from a blood sample were pending.

MANAGEMENT

- Patient was diagnosed with bilateral ICRB Group D Retinoblastoma.
- Patient underwent six cycles of vincristine + etoposide + carboplatin (VEC) therapy over a course of 4 months.
  - Side effects included a single event of low cell counts as well as fever, which necessitated hospitalization and IV antibiotic treatment.
- Adjuvant laser therapy (transpupillary thermotherapy [TTT] and cryotherapy) was performed four times in the right eye and twice in the left eye.

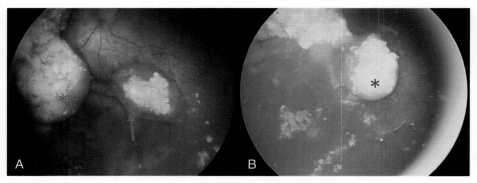

Fig. 47.2   (A) Right eye demonstrates a multifocal regressed mass of "cottage cheese" appearance *(red asterisk)*, with surrounding tumor with "fish-flesh" appearance *(red arrow)*. (B) Left eye demonstrates a regressed white, calcified mass *(blue asterisk)*.

FOLLOW-UP

- Genetic tests confirmed germ-line retinoblastoma.
- Last follow up at 45 months demonstrated a regressed, partially calcified tumor OD, with surrounding "fish flesh" appearance (Fig. 47.2A), while OS demonstrated a regressed white, calcified tumor (Fig.47.2B)
- Visual acuity was 20/400 OD and 20/30 OS.

KEY POINTS

- Management of bilateral medium-grade intraocular retinoblastoma is complex and may require the use of several treatment modalities.
- Historically, patients in these cases underwent bilateral enucleation, while modern centers today emphasize globe salvage, typically through chemoreduction combined with focal consolidation therapy (laser, cryotherapy, and plaque brachytherapy).
- Intravenous chemotherapy (IVC) combining vincristine + etoposide + carboplatin (VEC) is the most common regimen used today.
- IVC treatment can reduce the risk of metastatic disease and pinealoblastoma, as well as secondary neoplasms.
- Intra-arterial chemotherapy (IAC) has revolutionized the treatment of retinoblastoma by reducing IVC-related systemic toxicity, as well as improving ocular salvage rates, with various centers now incorporating simultaneous bilateral IAC therapy for bilateral disease.
- Intravitreal chemotherapy for intravitreal seeding compliments IVC and IAC in tumor control.
- Overall, regression patterns of retinoblastoma can be used to assess response to therapy, depending on extent of scar formation, calcification, and/or "fish-flesh" appearance.

CHAPTER 48

Retinoblastoma—Bilateral Advanced

Christine Ryu ■ Farid Khan ■ Aditya Maitray ■ Pukhraj Rishi

Strabismus in an 11-Month-Old Child

HISTORY OF PRESENT ILLNESS

A previously healthy 11-month-old male presents with large-angle esotropia of the right eye. Over the previous 2 months, the parents noted that the right eye has been turning in, initially intermittently but now appears to be stuck.

Exam

	OD	OS
External	Large-angle esotropia	Grossly orthotropic
Visual acuity	No fix, no follow	Fix and follow
IOP (mm Hg)	14	8
Sclera/conjunctiva	White and quiet	White and quiet
Cornea	Clear	Clear
AC	Deep, 1+ cell, neovascularization of the angle sparing 1 quadrant	Deep and quiet
Iris	Round and reactive, fine neovascularization	Round and reactive, no NVI
Lens	Clear	Clear
Vitreous	Clear	Vitreous cells
Optic nerve	Obscured by retinal mass	Mass abutting nerve, vitreous seeds overlying nerve (Fig. 48.1)
Retina	Retinal mass and total exudative retinal detachment	Mostly exophytic retinal mass involving macula

AC, Anterior chamber; *IOP,* intraocular pressure; *NVI,* neovascularization of the iris.

QUESTIONS TO ASK

- Has there been any white pupillary reflex in photos?
- Has anyone in the family been diagnosed with retinoblastoma? Is there any family history of blindness, eye disease requiring enucleation, or other childhood cancers?

The parents state that the eyes appear about the same in photos. On review of photos, there is bilateral, asymmetric leukocoria that is more prominent in the right eye (Fig. 48.2). Neither one

No financial interest associated with the manuscript. No funding supports.

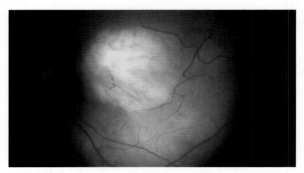

Fig. 48.1 Fundus photograph of left eye with Group D retinoblastoma. The tumor occupies the macula and abuts the optic nerve. The mass is mostly exophytic with a smaller, central, endophytic component. Vitreous seeds are seen over the optic nerve.

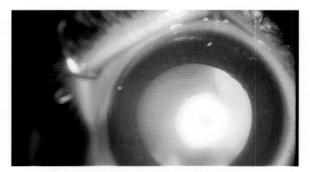

Fig. 48.2 Right eye with ICRB Group E retinoblastoma.

of the parents nor anyone else in the family has had retinoblastoma. Family history is negative for blindness, eye disease requiring enucleation, or other childhood cancers.

ASSESSMENT

- Total exudative retinal detachment, OD
- Neovascularization of angle, OD
- Retinal mass, OS

DIFFERENTIAL DIAGNOSIS

- Retinoblastoma
- Persistent fetal vasculature
- Retinopathy of prematurity
- Toxocariasis
- Vitreoretinal dysplasia

WORKING DIAGNOSIS

- Retinoblastoma, Intraocular Classification of Retinoblastoma (ICRB) Group E, OD
- Retinoblastoma, ICRB Group D, OS

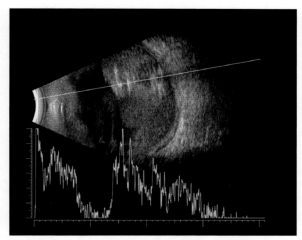

Fig. 48.3 B-scan of right eye with ICRB Group E retinoblastoma. A large hyperechoic mass occupies most of the vitreous cavity. Calcification is seen as hyperreflective foci with high amplitude and acoustic shadowing.

INVESTIGATION AND TESTING

- B-scan ultrasound of OD (Fig. 48.3) revealed a large, mixed, endophytic–exophytic mass occupying most of the vitreous cavity. Calcific foci with acoustic shadows were present. A-scan showed high internal reflectivity.
- B-scan ultrasound of OS revealed a posterior exophytic mass measuring 11.1 mm × 8.3 mm × 5.8 mm.
- MRI of orbits and brain with and without contrast did not reveal extraocular extension of the retinoblastoma in either eye. The optic nerves appeared normal in thickness, with no evidence of pinealoblastoma.

MANAGEMENT

- Group E retinoblastoma, OD
  - Primary enucleation with 13 mm segment of optic nerve. A polymethyl methacrylate orbital implant was placed.
  - Histopathology confirmed retinoblastoma with small, round, blue cells (Fig. 48.4A). The tumor was a mixed, endophytic–exophytic retinoblastoma occupying most of the posterior segment, draped by a total retinal detachment. The retrolaminar nerve was infiltrated (Fig. 48.4B), but the optic nerve margin was negative. Tumor cells were also found in the anterior chamber (Fig. 48.4C). There was choroidal extension of the retinoblastoma (Fig. 48.4D), but no invasion of the sclera.
  - Six cycles of adjuvant systemic chemotherapy with vincristine + etoposide + carboplatin (VEC) were initiated.
  - Referral to ocularist for ocular prosthesis.
- Group D retinoblastoma, OS
  - Given less severe presentation than the fellow eye, globe-sparing therapy was initiated with six cycles of systemic chemotherapy with VEC.
  - Significant regression of the tumor was noted on systemic chemotherapy, which was followed up with focal consolidation with transpupillary thermotherapy. The tumor and subretinal seeds regressed completely (Fig. 48.5).

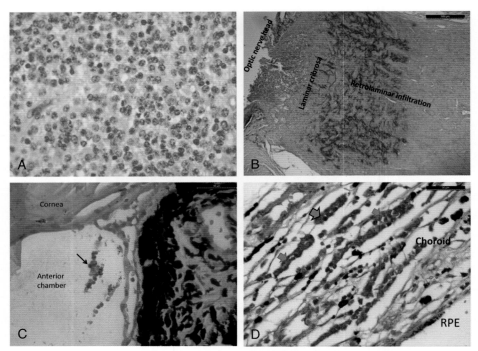

Fig. 48.4 (A) Histopathologic examination of enucleated right eye (H&E stain) demonstrates small, round, blue, hyperchromatic cells with scant cytoplasm that are packed into sheets and nests. (B) Invasion of the retinoblastoma cells seen in the retrolaminar optic nerve *(blue arrow)*, (C) anterior chamber *(black arrow)*, and (D) choroid *(blue arrows)*.

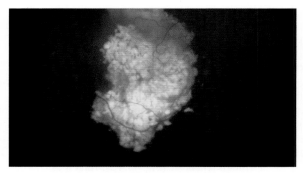

Fig. 48.5 Fundus photograph of the left eye after four cycles of systemic intravenous chemotherapy. The tumor has significantly reduced with type 3 regression.

FOLLOW-UP

- Exams under anesthesia (EUAs) initially every 4 weeks to monitor regression of tumor and subretinal seeding OS, then every 8 weeks until the age of 3
- MRI of orbits and brain with and without contrast every 6 months until the age of 5
- Lifelong routine eye exams, at least annually
- Lifelong monitoring for second cancers

KEY POINTS

- Retinoblastoma is the most common intraocular malignancy in children with an incidence of 250–300 cases per year in the United States. At presentation, about 40% of cases are bilateral.

- Transpupillary thermotherapy, cryotherapy, plaque brachytherapy, intraarterial chemotherapy, intravitreal chemotherapy, systemic chemotherapy, enucleation, and any combination of the above are used to treat retinoblastoma. External beam radiation therapy is no longer commonly used in view of the risk of second cancers.

- In cases of bilateral advanced retinoblastoma (Group D or E), globe salvage is attempted. The exception is concern for extraocular extension, in which case the eye is enucleated. Therapy can be initiated with either systemic chemotherapy (vincristine + etoposide + carboplatin [VEC]) or intraarterial chemotherapy (melphalan, carboplatin, or topotecan). Intravitreal chemotherapy with melphalan ± topotecan can also be used, especially for resistant vitreous seeds.

- Adjuvant therapy with systemic chemotherapy is considered when pathology after enucleation confirms intraocular containment of the tumor but with higher-risk findings. Higher-risk features include choroidal invasion ≥3 mm, retrolaminar optic nerve invasion with clean margins, and any combination of choroidal and optic nerve involvement.

- When pathology confirms that residual tumor is present after enucleation, such as transscleral invasion or tumor at optic nerve margin, systemic chemotherapy and orbital external beam radiation therapy are used.

CHAPTER 49

Retinoblastoma—Family History

Aurora Rodriguez ■ Todd Abruzzo ■ Aparna Ramasubramanian

Third-Generation Child With Bilateral Retinoblastoma

HISTORY OF PRESENT ILLNESS

A 3-year-old female with bilateral retinoblastoma presents for routine exam under anesthesia. Patient has been previously treated with systemic chemotherapy, intraarterial chemotherapy in both eyes, intravitreal chemotherapy in the left eye, and local treatment in both eyes. The family wants to know about the risks to their next child and the options available.

Exam

	OD	OS
IOP (mm Hg)	12	14
Anterior segment	Normal	Normal
Posterior segment	Normal vitreous	Normal vitreous
	Normal optic nerve	Normal optic nerve
	Regressed macular tumor, regressed peripheral seeds	Regressed macular tumor, regressed peripheral seeds

AC, Anterior chamber.

QUESTIONS TO ASK

- When was the child first diagnosed?
- Is there any history of cancer in the family?
- Has the child undergone genetic testing?

The child was diagnosed with bilateral retinoblastoma at 1 month old. Family history is positive for malignancy. Mother had bilateral retinoblastoma and osteosarcoma; maternal grandmother had bilateral retinoblastoma, nasopharyngeal carcinoma, and thyroid carcinoma. The genetic mutation has been identified in the child, mother, and maternal grandmother.

ASSESSMENT

- Bilateral familial retinoblastoma
- Family history of retinoblastoma and second cancers

No financial interest associated with the manuscript. No funding supports.

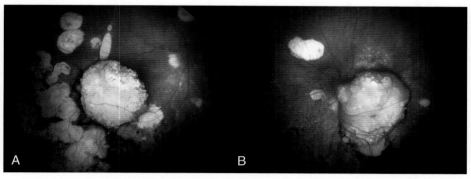

Fig. 49.1 Fundus photography shows regressed retinoblastoma tumors in (A) Right eye (B) Left eye.

WORKING DIAGNOSIS

- Familial bilateral retinoblastoma
- Genetic counseling for family

INVESTIGATION AND TESTING

- Fundus photography (Fig. 49.1)

MANAGEMENT

- Continue monitoring of child for relapse
- Genetic counseling and presentation of options to family:
  - Preimplantation testing
  - Early pregnancy testing
  - Late pregnancy testing

KEY POINTS

- Heritable retinoblastomas have an autosomal inheritance pattern. A child born to a parent with heritable retinoblastoma has a 45% chance of inheriting a germline mutated *Rb* allele due to 90% penetrance. Tumorigenesis relies on acquisition of somatic loss of function mutation in second copy of the gene.
- Early screening and diagnosis are important for a favorable prognosis. Options for screening include:
  - Prenatal screening
    - Preimplantation screening
    - Genetic testing is performed on embryos facilitated with in vitro fertilization; tests for *RB* gene mutations and other chromosomal abnormalities prior to embryo transfer (Fig. 49.2)
  - Early pregnancy screening
    - Chorionic villus sampling: partial removal and analysis of chorionic tissue under sonography guidance; safe to do after 10 weeks' gestation

Preimplantation Genetic Testing

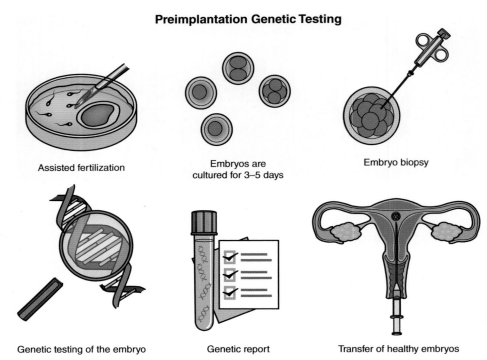

Fig. 49.2 Visual diagram representing the Preimplantation Genetic Testing process.

- Amniocentesis: partial extraction and analysis of amniotic fluid; can be done at 15 weeks' gestation
- Percutaneous umbilical cord sampling: fetal blood sampling via insertion of a needle into umbilical cord at 18–23 weeks
- Late pregnancy screening
  - Prenatal ultrasounds every 2 weeks starting at 32 weeks; fetal MRI may add to diagnostic evaluation at experienced centers; if antenatal diagnosis of retinoblastoma is confirmed, delivery is planned as early as possible after lung maturity is reached at 36 weeks to facilitate initiation of treatment as soon as possible
- Postnatal screening
  - Immediate genetic testing following the birth of the child, and after pretest risk of retinoblastoma is assessed; newborn also undergoes visual examination and optical coherence tomography (OCT) to look for occult tumors
  - Frequency and schedule for postnatal visual screenings based on pretest risk of retinoblastoma (Table 49.1)
  - Screening terminated after genetic testing with negative result

TABLE 49.1 ■ Pretest Risk of Retinoblastoma and Postnatal Screening Schedule Based on Risk Assessment

Postnatal Retinoblastoma Screening

	Pretest Risk of Retinoblastoma	
Relative of Proband	Bilateral Proband	Unilateral Proband
Offspring	50	7.5
Parent	5	0.8
Sibling	2.5	0.4
Niece/nephew	1.3	0.2
Aunt/uncle	0.1	0.007
First cousin	0.05	0.007
General population	0.007	

High Risk of Retinoblastoma ≥7.5	
Age	Screening
Birth–8 weeks	Every 2 weeks
8–12 weeks	Monthly
3–12 months	Monthly
12–24 months	Every 2 months
2–3 years	Every 3 months
3–4 years	Every 4 months
4–5 years	Every 6 months
5–7 years	Every 6 months

Intermediate Risk of Retinoblastoma 1–7.5	
Age	Screening
Birth–8 weeks	Monthly
8–12 weeks	Monthly
3–12 months	Every 2 months
12–24 months	Every 3 months
2–3 years	Every 3 months
3–4 years	Every 4 months
4–5 years	Every 6 months
5–7 years	Every 6 months

Low Risk of Retinoblastoma ≤1	
Age	Screening
Birth–8 weeks	Monthly
8–12 weeks	Monthly
3–12 months	Every 3 months
12–24 months	Every 4 months
2–3 years	Every 6 months
3–4 years	Every 6 months
4–5 years	Annually
5–7 years	Annually

Data from A. Skalet. (2017). "Screening children at risk for retinoblastoma: Consensus Report from the American Association of Ophthalmic Oncologists and Pathologists". *Ophthalmology*, 125(3), pp. 453–458. Copyright 2017 by Elsevier.

CHAPTER 50

Retinoblastoma—Orbital Involvement

Alejandra Etulain González ■ Jocelyn Lugo

Leukocoria and Decreased Visual Acuity in a 1-Year-Old Child

HISTORY OF PRESENT ILLNESS

A 1-year-old male presented with proptosis, pain, and redness of the right eye for 3 weeks. He had undergone surgery in both eyes for "congenital glaucoma" 2 months prior to presentation.

Exam

	OD	OS
Visual acuity	No light perception	Fixes briefly
IOP (mm Hg)	35	9
Sclera/conjunctiva	Conjunctival congestion	Conjunctival bleb
Cornea	Hazy (Fig. 50.1)	Clear
AC	No view	Deep and quiet
Iris	No view	Unremarkable
		Brown iris, pupil round
		No NVI
Lens	No view	Clear
Anterior vitreous	No view	Clear
Retina/optic nerve	No view	Clear

AC, Anterior chamber; *IOP,* intraocular pressure; *NVI,* neovascularization of the iris.

QUESTIONS TO ASK

- Is there a previous history of redness or pain in the eye?
- Is there any history of cancer in the family?
- Does the child have any other relevant medical history?

The mother reports that 6 months earlier she had noticed that the child had a white spot on the eye, and the eye began to become big and red after that. The child was diagnosed with congenital glaucoma and underwent trabeculectomy in both eyes. There is no history of cancer in the family and the child has no other significant past medical history.

No financial interest associated with the manuscript. No funding supports.

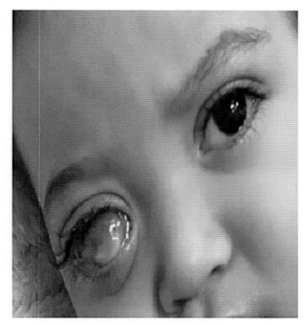

Fig. 50.1 Accidental orbital retinoblastoma. Trabeculectomy in both eyes in an eye with unsuspected retino-blastoma in a 1-year-old male.

ASSESSMENT

- Proptosis
- Previous trabeculotomy, OU

DIFFERENTIAL DIAGNOSIS

- Orbital retinoblastoma
- Rhabdomyosarcoma
- Lymphoma
- Ewing sarcoma

WORKING DIAGNOSIS

- Orbital retinoblastoma, OD

INVESTIGATION AND TESTING

- Magnetic resonance of the orbits and brain showed a calcified intraocular tumor in the right eye with diffuse soft-tissue thickening around the eye (Fig. 50.2).
- Bone marrow biopsy was negative to neoplastic cells.
- Cerebrospinal fluid cytology was negative to neoplastic cells.
- Bone scintigraphy with Tc-99m showed no osteoblastic activity.

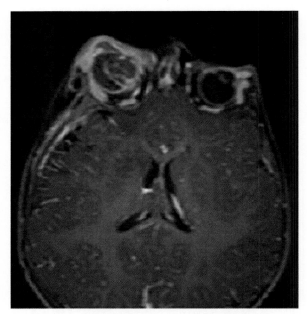

Fig. 50.2 Magnetic resonance image showing intraocular tumor occupying the entire vitreous cavity and diffuse soft-tissue thickening around the eye.

- PET scan showed evidence of exophytic ocular neoplasia with extraocular involvement of soft tissues and skin of the upper eyelid, which infiltrates the superior and lateral rectus muscles of the right orbit as well as the lacrimal gland.

MANAGEMENT

- Initial high-dose chemotherapy with carboplatin, ifosfamide, and etoposide for four cycles every 21 days
- Followed by modified (enlarged) enucleation right eye
- External-beam radiation therapy to orbit and cervical nodes (45 Gy fractionated)
- Additional two cycles of high-dose adjuvant chemotherapy

FOLLOW-UP

- Pathology of the enucleated globe showed massive infiltration of the choroid, ciliary bodies, anterior chamber, cornea, sclera, and adjacent soft tissue (Fig. 50.3). The optic nerve (length: 11 mm) showed postlaminar invasion with no involvement of cut section of optic nerve (Figs. 50.4 and 50.5).
- The patient is in the first year following treatment and continues to do well with periodic examination under anesthesia and MRI every 3 months.

KEY POINTS

- Orbital retinoblastoma can be classified as followed:
  - Primary orbital retinoblastoma—orbital extension at initial presentation

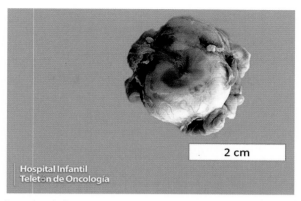

Fig. 50.3 Collapsed eyeball measuring 2.5 cm × 2 cm × 2.2 cm with adhesions on the sclera.

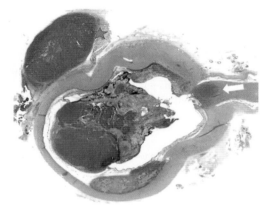

Fig. 50.4 Histological section (H&E stain) with invasion of soft tissues *(green star)* and retrolaminar invasion of optic nerve >1 mm *(white arrow)*.

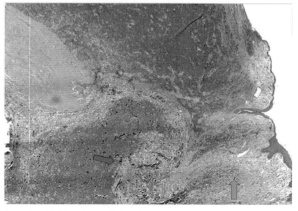

Fig. 50.5 Histological section (H&E stain, 40x) showing ciliary body invasion *(red arrow)* and diffuse invasion of anterior chamber and cornea *(blue arrow)*.

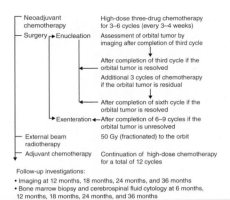

High-dose chemotherapy:

Vincristine, 0.025 mg/kg, day 1 / Etoposide, 12 mg/kg, days 1 and 2 / carboplatin, 28 mg/kg, day 1

Fig. 50.6 Treatment protocol for orbital retinoblastoma. (*Data from Honavar SG Manjandavida FP, Reddy VP. Orbital retionblastoma: An update. Indian J Ophthalmol 2017;65:435–442.*)

- Secondary orbital retinoblastoma—orbital recurrence following primary treatment
- Accidental orbital retinoblastoma—inadvertent perforation during enucleation, fine-needle aspiration biopsy, or intraocular surgery in an eye with unsuspected intraocular retinoblastoma
- Overt orbital retinoblastoma—extrascleral or optic nerve extension discovered during enucleation
- Microscopic orbital retinoblastoma—full-thickness scleral infiltration, extrascleral extension, or invasion of cut end of optic nerve seen on pathology after enucleation
- Treatment for orbital retinoblastoma is complex and requires multimodal management with a combination of chemotherapy, surgery, and radiotherapy.
- Honavar et al.[1] developed a treatment protocol comprising initial triple-drug high-dose chemotherapy (vincristine + etoposide + carboplatin [VEC]) for three to six cycles every 21–28 days, followed by appropriate surgery (enucleation, extended enucleation, or orbital exenteration), orbital radiotherapy (50 Gy fractionated) to the orbit, and complete chemotherapy for a total of 12 cycles, also of high-dose chemotherapy (Fig. 50.6). With this protocol, authors reported a dramatic resolution of orbital involvement and a mean event-free survival of 36 months in 90% of patients.

Reference

1. Honavar SG, Manjandavida FP, Reddy VP. Orbital retinoblastoma: An update. *Indian J Ophthalmol.* 2017;65:435–442.

CHAPTER 51

Retinoblastoma—Metastatic

Thanaporn Kritfuangfoo ■ Ratima Chokchaitanasin ■ Wantanee Dangboon
Tsutsumi ■ Duangnate Rojanaporn

Leukocoria, Neovascular Glaucoma, and Subconjunctival Mass in a 20-Month-Old Male

HISTORY OF PRESENT ILLNESS

A 20-month-old healthy male presents with leukocoria and red eye OS. His mother noticed that the child cannot see well, as he often hit objects and has fallen over the past 6 months. His mother also noticed a red eye with white pupil in the left eye. He has no prior traumatic events or ocular illness.

Exam

	OD	OS
Visual acuity	Can fix and follow	Cannot fix and follow
IOP (mm Hg)	8	43
Sclera/conjunctiva	White and quiet	Ciliary injection with subconjunctival mass (Fig. 51.1)
Cornea	Clear	Hazy
AC	Deep and quiet	Dense whitish cellular aggregation in AC (Fig. 51.2A)
Iris	Unremarkable Brown iris, round pupil with no NVI	NVI
Lens	Clear	Clear
Vitreous	Clear	Dense vitreous haziness
Retina/optic nerve	Normal	Obscured fundus

AC, Anterior chamber; *IOP,* intraocular pressure; *NVI,* neovascularization of the iris.

QUESTIONS TO ASK

■ Is there any history of cancer in the family?
■ Does the child have any other relevant past medical history?
■ Does the child have any other systemic symptoms?

There is no ocular or systemic cancer in his family. There was no significant medical history. The child has no other systemic symptoms.

No financial interest associated with the manuscript. No funding supports.

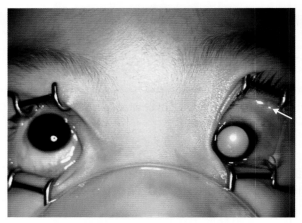

Fig. 51.1 External photograph shows leukocoria, ciliary injection, and subconjunctival mass *(white arrow)* in the left eye.

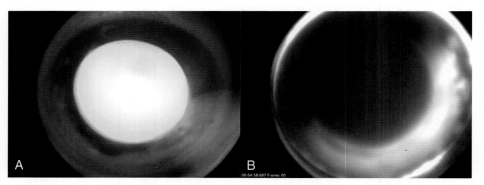

Fig. 51.2 (A) The anterior segment photograph of the left eye shows corneal edema with white tumor cell aggregates in the anterior chamber. (B) Anterior segment fluorescein angiography shows iris neovascularization.

ASSESSMENT

- Leukocoria, OS
- Neovascular glaucoma, OS
- Subconjunctival mass, OS
- Vitreous haziness, OS
- Anterior chamber seeding, OS

DIFFERENTIAL DIAGNOSIS

- Retinoblastoma
- Orbital cellulitis
- Endophthalmitis
- Coats disease

WORKING DIAGNOSIS

- Extraocular retinoblastoma, OS

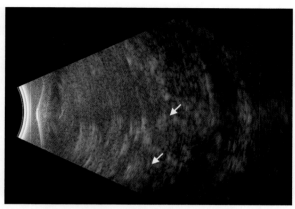

Fig. 51.3   B-scan ultrasonography shows hyperechoic mass occupying the entire globe with multiple calcium deposits, seen as hyperechoic foci *(white arrows)*.

INVESTIGATION AND TESTING

- Fluorescein angiography of the left eye shows iris neovascularization (Fig. 51.2B).
- B-scan ultrasonography of the left eye shows a large hyperechoic mass occupying the entire globe with multiple calcium deposits, seen as hyperechoic foci (Fig. 51.3).
- MRI scans of the brain and orbits showed an intraocular mass occupying nearly the entire left globe and extending along the intraorbital and intracanalicular segments of the left optic nerve. There is extraocular extension as a subconjunctival mass. The brain and right globe are unremarkable (Fig. 51.4A).
- A lumbar puncture and bone marrow aspiration were performed to evaluate for the presence of metastatic disease, and there was no evidence of tumor cells.

MANAGEMENT

- The treatment of extraocular retinoblastoma often involves a combination therapy, which has been shown to be more effective. The treatment typically begins with systemic chemotherapy administered over three to six cycles, followed by surgery, which may include enucleation, extended enucleation, or orbital exenteration, as appropriate. Additional chemotherapy or radiotherapy is determined based on the results of the residual tumor after surgical removal and the pathological examination.
- In this patient, the pediatric oncologist administered a high-dose systemic chemotherapy regimen consisting of vincristine + etoposide + carboplatin (VEC) (Table 51.1). The MRI was performed to evaluate the tumor response after every three cycles of chemotherapy.

FOLLOW-UP

- The tumor failed to respond to high-dose chemotherapy. After three cycles of high-dose chemotherapy, subsequent MRI scans revealed an increase in size of the intraocular tumor and extraocular extension along the left optic nerve, left-sided optic chiasm, and anterior aspect of the left optic tract (Fig. 51.4B).
- During the course of treatment, the patient developed leptomeningeal metastasis along the bilateral cerebral and cerebellar sulci (Fig. 51.4C), as well as spinal metastasis (Fig. 51.4D).
- At the end of treatment, the patient developed status epilepticus and alteration of consciousness, and he passed away a few weeks later.

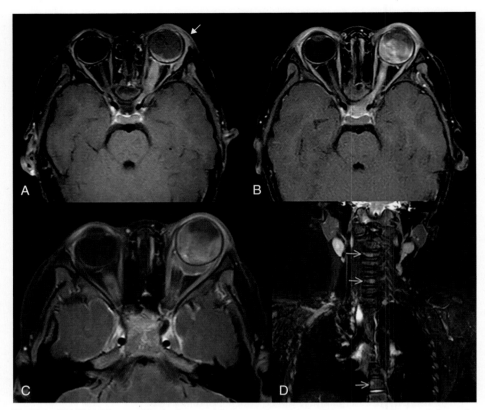

Fig. 51.4 (A) Initial MRI scan of the brain and orbit shows a large intraocular mass occupying nearly the entire left globe with extraocular involvement in the area of subconjunctival mass *(white arrow)*, intraorbital, and intracanalicular segment of the left optic nerve. (B) A subsequent MRI scan following high-dose systemic chemotherapy shows progression of intraocular tumor size, with extraocular extension along the left optic nerve, optic chiasm, and anterior aspect of the left optic tract. (C) The patient developed leptomeningeal metastasis along the bilateral cerebral and cerebellar sulci, and (D) spinal metastasis *(green arrows)*.

TABLE 51.1 ■ **Chemotherapy Regimen for Extraocular Extension and Metastatic Retinoblastoma in Children's Oncology Group Trial (ARET0321)**

	Systemic Chemotherapy	
Extraocular extension	Carboplatin	28 mg/kg/day on day 1
	Etoposide	12 mg/kg/day on days 1–2
	Vincristine	0.025 mg/kg/day on day 1
Metastatic retinoblastoma	Carboplatin	18.7 mg/kg or 560 mg/m^2/day on day 1
	Ifosfamide[a]	60 mg/kg or 1,800 mg/m^2/day on days 1–5
	Etoposide	3.3 mg/kg or 100 mg/m^2/day on days 1–5
	MTX, Ara-C	Intrathecal chemotherapy for CNS involvement

CNS, Central nervous involvement.
[a]Hydration following high-dose ifosfamide guideline.

KEY POINTS

- Retinoblastoma can manifest as uveitis, neovascular glaucoma, or orbital cellulitis.
- MRI has an invaluable role in disease staging, as well as evaluating treatment response.
- Metastasis is an important cause of death in patients with retinoblastomas. The frequency of metastatic retinoblastoma in developing countries is approximately 10%.
- The most common metastatic site of retinoblastoma is the CNS, accounting for approximately 50% of cases. Optic nerve involvement is the most important risk factor for CNS metastasis. The bone is the second most common site.
- The multimodal treatment for metastatic retinoblastoma includes intensive systemic chemotherapy with autologous hematopoietic stem cells rescue, combined fractionated radiotherapy, and intrathecal chemotherapy (Table 51.1).

CHAPTER 52

Retinoblastoma—Second Malignancy

Sarah Zhang ■ Lindsey Hoffman

Osteosarcoma Secondary to *RB1* Germline Mutation

PRESENTING ILLNESS

Shoulder pain in an 18-year-old patient with germline *RB1* mutation.

HISTORY OF PRESENT ILLNESS

An 18-year-old male with germline *RB1* mutation presents with new left shoulder pain. The patient reported mild pain when lifting weights starting 4 months ago. He was referred to physical therapy and used topical anesthetic gels and oral nonsteroidal antiinflammatory medications without relief. The pain continued to increase, so he presented to the emergency department for additional workup.

PAST MEDICAL HISTORY

Bilateral retinoblastoma at age 7 months. He received six cycles of systemic chemotherapy followed by focal proton beam radiation therapy to the left eye.

PAST SURGICAL HISTORY

- Enucleation of right eye
- Central line placement and removal

FAMILY HISTORY

No family history of retinoblastoma (*de novo* germline mutation in affected patient).

Exam

	OD	OS
Visual acuity	Anophthalmos	20/60
IOP (mm Hg)	Anophthalmos	15
Sclera/conjunctiva	Anophthalmos	Normal
Cornea	Anophthalmos	Punctate keratitis

No financial interest associated with the manuscript. No funding supports.

Exam—cont'd

	OD	OS
AC	Anophthalmos	Normal
Iris	Anophthalmos	Normal
Lens	Anophthalmos	Horizontal linear posterior subcapsular cataract
Anterior vitreous	Anophthalmos	Clear
Retina/optic nerve	Anophthalmos	Mild pallor optic nerve
		Macular scar, all peripheral tumors regressed

AC, Anterior chamber; *IOP,* intraocular pressure.

HEENT: Normocephalic, nose and oropharynx clear, moist mucous membranes
Cardiovascular: Regular rate and rhythm; no murmurs, rubs, gallops; cap refill <3 seconds; no edema
Lungs: Normal work of breathing; lungs clear to auscultation bilaterally
Abdomen: Soft, nontender, nondistended, no hepatosplenomegaly or masses
Skin: Warm, dry, no rashes; small scar noted on right chest wall from prior central line
Neurology: Alert and oriented, grossly normal strength and sensation; CN II–XII grossly intact
Musculoskeletal: Pain with abduction of left shoulder; palpable mass and tenderness over proximal left upper extremity; no pain with movement of any other joints
Lymph: No cervical lymphadenopathy
Psych: Normal mood and affect

QUESTIONS TO ASK

- What treatments did you have for retinoblastoma?
- Did you have any recent injuries or trauma?
- Do you have any weight loss?
- Do you have any redness or swelling?

The patient had no history of injury, redness, or swelling to his left shoulder. He had previously received radiation therapy to his right orbit as treatment for retinoblastoma as an infant, but his left shoulder was not in the radiation field. He had mild fatigue recently but no weight loss or other systemic symptoms.

ASSESSMENT

- Left shoulder pain and mass in a patient with germline *RB1* mutation

DIFFERENTIAL DIAGNOSIS

- Metastatic relapse of retinoblastoma
- Primary malignancy associated with *RB1* germline loss: osteosarcoma or melanoma
- Benign bone tumors: osteoblastoma, osteoid osteoma, chondroma
- Nonneoplastic conditions: osteomyelitis, septic arthritis, aneurysmal bone cysts

WORKING DIAGNOSIS

- Osteosarcoma as second primary malignancy associated with *RB1*

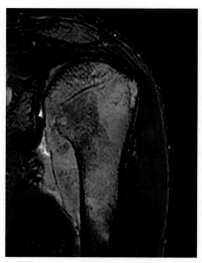

Fig. 52.1 MRI left shoulder with and without contrast showing large heterogeneous intramedullary lesion within the left humeral head and neck with destruction of the medial bony cortex and soft tissue extension just inferior to the glenoid.

INVESTIGATION AND TESTING

- MRI of left shoulder revealed a heterogeneous tumor involving the humeral head and proximal humerus (Fig. 52.1).
- PET CT scan of the whole body showed increased metabolic uptake of the left humerus with no other obvious sites of metastatic disease (Fig. 52.2).

MANAGEMENT

- The patient underwent a biopsy of the tumor, which confirmed osteoblastic osteosarcoma.
- The patient underwent chemotherapy followed by primary tumor resection. At the time of resection, 99% of the tumor was necrotic (a good prognostic sign) (Fig. 52.3).

FOLLOW-UP

- The patient completed therapy and underwent chest CT scan and MRI of the left shoulder every 3 months for the first year and every 6 months for the second year off therapy with no evidence of disease recurrence.

KEY POINTS

- Approximately 33.1% of hereditary retinoblastoma survivors at 50 years develop a subsequent malignant neoplasm (SMN) with a median age of 15–17.
- Heritable retinoblastoma survivors treated with radiotherapy are at a 3.1-fold greater risk of developing SMN than those not treated with radiotherapy.
- There is especially increased risk of developing osteosarcoma (36.4%), soft-tissue sarcoma (11.5%), melanoma (8%), and brain tumors (4%).

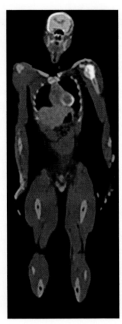

Fig. 52.2 PET CT scan shows area of increased metabolic activity involving the proximal left humerus with no evidence of metastatic disease.

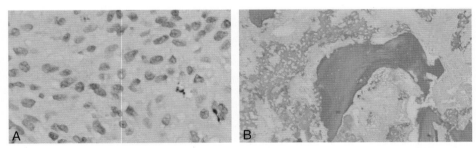

Fig. 52.3 (A) Histology of the osteoblastic osteosarcoma biopsy specimen at 400x magnification demonstrating cytologic atypia and high mitotic activity. (B) Posttreatment specimen at 40x magnification demonstrates necrotic tissue with rare viable atypical cells.

- There is evidence that radiotherapy plus an alkylating chemotherapy increase the risks for leiomyosarcoma and bone tumors compared to radiotherapy alone.
- Due to the increased risk of developing SMN, surveillance recommendations for retinoblastoma survivors include annual skin exam, patient and physician education on SMNs, prompt medical evaluation for any new concerns, and participation in national cancer surveillance programs.

CHAPTER 53

Pinealoblastoma

Aurora Rodriguez ■ Jocelyn Juarez ■ Alejandra Etulain González
■ Aparna Ramasubramanian

7-Month-Old Child With Bilateral Retinoblastoma and Pinealoblastoma

HISTORY OF PRESENT ILLNESS

A 7-month-old female presented with esotropia and bilateral leukocoria. The child was born full term and did not have any other significant medical history.

Exam

	OD	OS
Visual acuity	Brief fix	No fix or follow
IOP (mm Hg)	15	25
Sclera/conjunctiva	White and quiet	Mild congestion
Cornea	Clear	Clear
AC	Deep and quiet	Deep and quiet
Iris	Unremarkable	NVI
	Brown iris, pupil round, no NVI	
Lens	Clear	Clear
Anterior vitreous	Clear	Clear
Retina/optic nerve	Three elevated retinal tumors obstructing the majority of the vitreous cavity	Elevated retinal tumor occupying most of the vitreous cavity (Fig. 53.1B)
	Vitreous seeds also present (Fig. 53.1A)	

AC, Anterior chamber; *IOP,* intraocular pressure; *NVI,* neovascularization of the iris.

QUESTIONS TO ASK

■ Is there any history of cancer in the family?
■ Is the child developmentally normal?

There is no family history of malignancy. The child's growth and development have been normal since birth.

ASSESSMENT

■ Bilateral retinoblastoma

No financial interest associated with the manuscript. No funding supports.

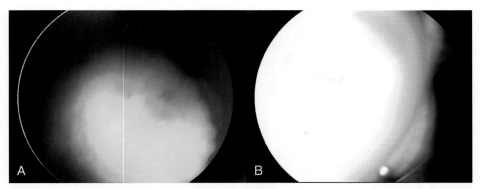

Fig. 53.1 Fundus photography shows retinoblastoma tumors in both eyes. (A) OD corresponds to 1A. (B) OS corresponds to 1B.

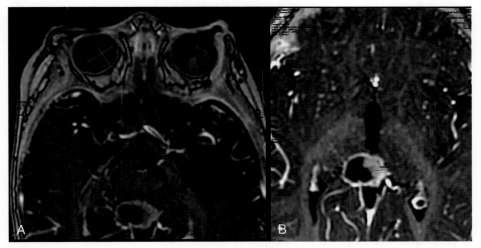

Fig. 53.2 MRI imaging with contrast. (A) Bilateral intraocular retinoblastoma with no signs of optic nerve or choroidal invasion. (B) Pineal tumor with solid and cystic components.

DIFFERENTIAL DIAGNOSIS

- Pineal cyst
- Pinealoblastoma

WORKING DIAGNOSIS

- Bilateral retinoblastoma: OD group D, OS group E

INVESTIGATION AND TESTING

- MRI with contrast showed bilateral intraocular retinoblastoma with no signs of optic nerve or choroidal invasion (Fig. 53.2A) and a 12.4 mm × 18.3 mm × 18.6 mm pineal tumor with solid and cystic components (Fig. 53.2B).
- Lumbar puncture and bone marrow biopsy were negative.

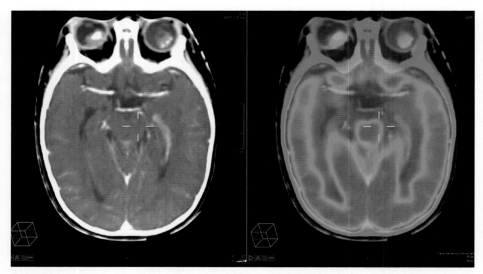

Fig. 53.3 PET scan imaging shows glycolytic metabolism consistent with neoplastic activity intraocularly and in the pineal gland.

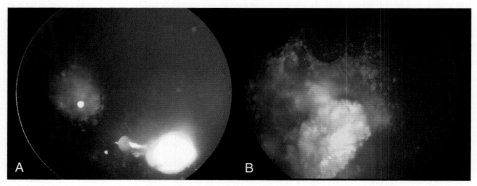

Fig. 53.4 Fundus photography shows regressed retinoblastoma tumors in both eyes. (A) OD corresponds to 4A. (B) OS corresponds to 4B.

- Genetic testing showed germline retinoblastoma mutation.
- PET scan showed metabolic activity only intraocularly and in the pineal region (Fig. 53.3).

MANAGEMENT

- Patient underwent four cycles of alternative induction treatment with high-dose chemotherapy and stem-cell harvest. This was followed by consolidation therapy according to the ARET0321 advanced 4b tumor protocol.
- Following completion of chemotherapy, the patient underwent four sessions of localized laser photocoagulation to the right eye.

FOLLOW-UP

- Patient is being monitored for tumor regression and relapse.
- The intraocular tumors have remained regressed (Fig. 53.4A–B).

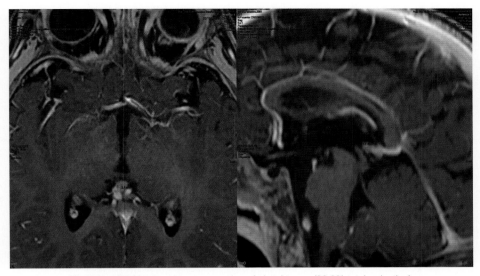

Fig. 53.5   MRI imaging shows regression of pineal tumor (99.3% total reduction).

- The pineal tumor has shown a good regression (Fig. 53.5), and the child's growth and development have been normal.

KEY POINTS

- Pinealoblastoma is a highly malignant, rare neoplasm arising from neuroectodermal cells in the pineal gland. The presence of a pineal gland tumor in the setting of bilateral retinoblastoma is termed "trilateral retinoblastoma."
- Pinealoblastomas have a poor prognosis. Thus, early diagnosis and implementation of treatment are crucial to improve the clinical outcome of the patient.
- The treatment of pinealoblastoma in the setting of bilateral retinoblastoma follows the ARET0321 stage 4b protocol (Children's Oncology Group Protocol), which is an Intensive Multi-Modality Therapy for Extra-Ocular Retinoblastoma.
  - The stage 4b protocol comprises an induction period followed by a consolidation phase of therapy.
    - Standard Chemotherapy Induction Regimen
      1. Consists of four cycles of vincristine, cyclophosphamide with mesna coadministration, carboplatin, and etoposide.
         - On day 3 of each cycle, the patient receives G-CSF until absolute neutrophil count (ANC) is equal or greater to 200.
      2. Patients who experience carboplatin-related hearing loss greater than 20 db at 500–400 Hz during treatment should switch to the alternative chemotherapy regimen for the remaining induction period.
    - Alternative Induction Chemotherapy Regimen
      1. Indicated for patients with preexisting ototoxicity or expected visual impairment.
      2. Consists of four cycles of chemotherapy. The initial two cycles are composed of vincristine, cyclophosphamide with mesna coadministration, and etoposide. The remaining two cycles consist of vincristine, carboplatin, and etoposide.
         - On day 3 of each cycle, the patient receives G-CSF until ANC is equal or greater to 200.

    3. For advanced tumors (stage 4a or 4b), the patient undergoes peripheral blood stem cell harvest between cycles 2 and 3.

- Consolidation Phase of Therapy
  1. Indicated only for those with advanced tumor disease (e.g., trilateral retinoblastoma).
  2. Consists of a multiday administration of carboplatin, thiotepa, and etoposide over 4–6 weeks.
  3. IV stem-cell infusion is indicated 48 hours after completing consolidation chemotherapy.

- Patients who have received chemoreduction require examinations under anesthesia. Usually, surveillance visits happen every 6–8 weeks until the age of 3 years. Children with germ-line mutations require long-term, special vigilance for tumor regression and secondary malignancies.

Nonpigmented Posterior Segment Tumors

CHAPTER 54

Choroid Metastasis—Isolated

Janelle Marie Fassbender Adeniran

Decreased Visual Acuity in a Woman With a History of Cancer

HISTORY OF PRESENT ILLNESS

A 74-year-old female presented with decreased vision in her right eye. She had noticed sudden worsening vision 2 weeks prior and sought care from her local optometrist. The optometrist referred her to a retinal specialist for evaluation of retinal detachment OD. She has no prior ocular history or trauma to either eye.

Exam

	OD	OS
Visual acuity	20/200	20/30
IOP (mm Hg)	9	10
Sclera/conjunctiva	White and quiet	White and quiet
Cornea	Clear	Clear
AC	Deep and quiet	Deep and quiet
Iris	Unremarkable	Unremarkable
Lens	2+ NS	2+ NS
Anterior vitreous	Clear, negative for pigment or cells	Clear, negative for pigment or cells
Retina/optic nerve	Normal optic nerve	Normal optic nerve
	16 mm × 14 mm, very elevated, amelanotic, choroidal mass with orange pigment and mild SRF overlying the lesion	2 mm × 2 mm mildly elevated, amelanotic, choroidal nodule on the temporal macula and smaller nodule outside the inferotemporal arcade

AC, Anterior chamber; *IOP,* intraocular pressure; *NS,* nuclear sclerosis; *SRF,* subretinal fluid.

QUESTIONS TO ASK

- Do you have any personal history of cancer?
- Is there any history of cancer in your family?
- Do you have any other relevant medical history?

The patient has triple-negative breast cancer, initially diagnosed in 2020, status post (s/p) chemotherapy and radiation with PET scan 2 months prior showing possible metastases versus new primary

No financial interest associated with the manuscript. No funding supports.

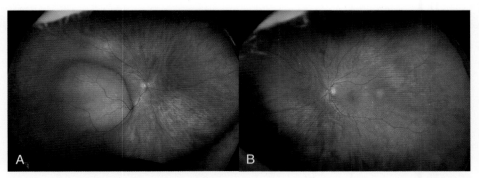

Fig. 54.1 Color fundus photos of (A) the right eye showing a dome-shaped amelanotic choroidal mass extending from the temporal equator to the fovea and (B) the left eye showing smaller but multifocal amelanotic lesions in the temporal macula and inferotemporal midperiphery.

metastasis in the lungs. She underwent a recent thoracentesis of the associated pleural effusion—the cytology is pending. The patient reports no known lesions to the brain.

ASSESSMENT

- Large, amelanotic choroidal mass, OD
- Small, multifocal, amelanotic choroidal masses, OS

DIFFERENTIAL DIAGNOSIS

- Choroidal metastasis
- Choroidal melanoma
- Choroidal granuloma

WORKING DIAGNOSIS

- Choroidal metastasis secondary to metastatic breast cancer, OU

INVESTIGATION AND TESTING

- Fundus color photography (Fig. 54.1)
- Fundus autofluorescence
- B-scan ultrasound (Fig. 54.2)
- Fluorescein angiogram

MANAGEMENT

- The patient underwent external beam radiation to all lesions and restarted systemic chemotherapy.

FOLLOW-UP

- Excellent regression was noted at 6 weeks following targeted external beam radiation (Fig. 54.3).

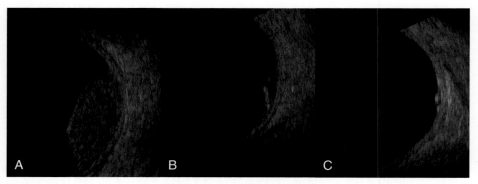

Fig. 54.2 Ultrasound demonstrating the dome-shaped choroidal mass in the right eye (A), smaller lesion in the temporal macula in the left eye (B), and even small lesion outside the inferotemporal arcade (C).

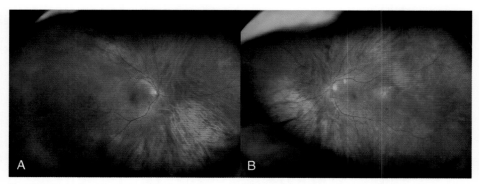

Fig. 54.3 Color fundus photo of (A) the right eye and (B) the left eye showing complete regression of the choroidal metastatic lesions at 6 weeks following external beam radiation and reinitiation of chemotherapy.

KEY POINTS

- Choroidal metastases are the most common intraocular cancers.
- The most common primary sites for choroidal metastases include the lung, breast, gastrointestinal tract, kidney, skin (melanoma), and prostate.
- Management may include systemic chemotherapy with targeted external beam irradiation, plaque brachytherapy, or photodynamic therapy. Choice of therapy may depend on the size, location, and number of lesions as well as the systemic status of the patient.
- The prognosis for patients with choroidal metastasis is variable depending on the type of cancer and the systemic disease burden.

CHAPTER 55

CHOROID METASTASIS— MULTIFOCAL

Mrittika Sen ▪ Carol L. Shields

Painless, Progressive Decreased Vision in the Right Eye of a 69-Year-Old Female With a Choroidal Lesion

HISTORY OF PRESENT ILLNESS

A 69-year-old White female presented with history of blurred vision OD for 4 months. She was referred with a retinal lesion in the right eye.

Exam

	OD	OS
Visual acuity	Counting fingers 3 feet	20/40
IOP (mm Hg)	15	17
Sclera/conjunctiva	White and quiet	White and quiet
Cornea	Clear	Clear
AC	Deep and quiet	Deep and quiet
Iris	Unremarkable	Unremarkable
	Blue iris, pupil round	Blue iris, pupil round
Lens	NS grade 1	NS grade 1
Anterior vitreous	Clear	Clear
Retina/optic nerve	Two discrete, yellow, choroidal lesions. The first lesion was 1 mm to disc and 0 mm to fovea and measured 10 mm × 10 mm × 3.3 mm with surrounding SRF. The second lesion was along the inferonasal arcade, 3 mm to disc, 6 mm to fovea, and measured 3 mm × 2 mm × 1.9 mm with no SRF and orange pigmentation.	Normal, cup disc ration 0.2, macula intact, retina attached

AC, Anterior chamber; *IOP,* intraocular pressure; *NS,* nuclear sclerosis; *SRF,* subretinal fluid.

Support provided in part by the Eye Tumor Research Foundation, Philadelphia, PA (CLS). The funders had no role in the design and conduct of the study; in the collection, analysis, and interpretation of the data; and in the preparation, review, or approval of the manuscript. Carol L. Shields, MD, has had full access to all the data in the study and takes responsibility for the integrity of the data.

QUESTIONS TO ASK

- Do you have any significant medical history?
- Is there any family history of cancer?

The patient was diagnosed 10 years ago with left-sided breast cancer with metastasis to lymph nodes and more recent relapse with right-sided breast cancer and biopsy-proven pleural and mediastinal metastases. She had undergone left mastectomy with lymph node dissection, chemotherapy, and external beam radiation 10 years ago. The oncologist had planned to reinitiate systemic chemotherapy for metastatic disease. There was also a family history of breast cancer in a first cousin.

ASSESSMENT

- Amelanotic multifocal choroidal lesions with subretinal fluid, OD
- History of metastatic breast cancer

DIFFERENTIAL DIAGNOSIS

- Choroid metastases, OD, multifocal
- Choroid melanoma, amelanotic, multifocal
- Choroid granuloma
- Choroidal lymphoma

WORKING DIAGNOSIS

- Choroid metastasis, OD, multifocal (Fig. 55.1)

INVESTIGATION AND TESTING

- B-scan ultrasound of OD showed an echodense choroidal lesion with medium internal reflectivity (Fig. 55.2).

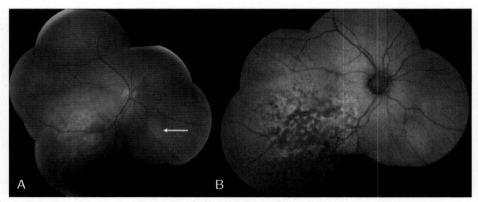

Fig. 55.1 Fundus photograph of the right eye showing (A) amelanotic, yellow, multifocal choroidal metastases from breast cancer. The macular lesion has associated subretinal fluid. The smaller lesion *(white arrow)* is more subtle with minimal elevation and no subretinal fluid. (B) The autofluorescence showing mixed hypo- and hyperautofluorescence.

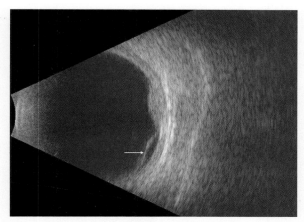

Fig. 55.2   B-scan ultrasound showing an echodense dome-shaped choroidal lesion with thickness 3.3 mm with subretinal fluid *(white arrow)*.

- Optical coherence tomography (OCT) showed an irregular lumpy configuration of the choroid with subretinal fluid (Fig. 55.3).

MANAGEMENT

- The options for management included external beam radiotherapy, plaque radiotherapy, photodynamic therapy, and systemic chemotherapy.
- Although systemic chemotherapy was already planned for the patient, the choroidal lesions required aggressive treatment, as they were likely to enlarge and further deteriorate her visual acuity.
- In view of the unilateral, multifocal nature of the metastasis and associated exudative retinal detachment, external beam radiotherapy with 4000 cGy to OD was preferred.
- Patient was referred to a radiation oncologist for the same and advised about long-term follow-up for systemic monitoring with the oncologist.

FOLLOW-UP

- The patient underwent external beam radiotherapy OD; however, she was lost to follow-up.

KEY POINTS

- The uveal tissue is the most common site of hematogenous ophthalmic metastasis owing to its rich blood supply, with lesions most commonly involving the choroid (90%), followed by the iris (8%) and ciliary body (2%).
- The mean age at diagnosis of ocular metastasis is 60 years (10–94 years) with breast cancer demonstrating a relatively younger age of presentation. Uveal metastasis is rare in children (<20 years) and senior adults (>80 years).
- Uveal metastasis is more common in females (64%) and unilateral (82%). The mean number of tumors per eye is 1.7. In females, uveal metastasis is most commonly from the breast, uterus, and ovary, and in males it is most commonly from the lung, esophagus, prostate, and stomach. Females also show a younger age of diagnosis, bilateral disease, and multifocal ocular metastasis as compared to males.

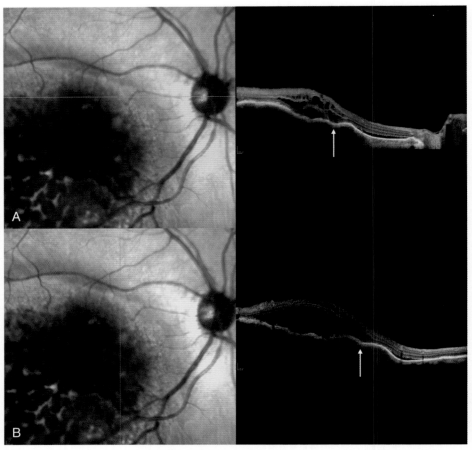

Fig. 55.3 Optical coherence tomography (OCT) through the fovea showing choroidal metastasis with (A) cystoid macular edema in the horizontal section and (B) subretinal fluid in the vertical section with a typical undulating, "lumpy-bumpy" choroidal contour *(white arrows)*.

- The mean time interval between diagnosis of primary tumor and uveal metastasis in patients with known primary is 5.2 years. Lung and gastrointestinal cancers have early onset of uveal metastasis, while breast and thyroid cancers have relatively late-onset uveal metastasis.
- On B-scan ultrasound, choroidal metastasis appears as an echodense dome-shaped or placoid lesion. On fluorescein angiography, it demonstrates early hyperfluorescence, multifocal retinal-pigment-epithelial pinpoint leaks, and late staining without the "double circulation" seen in uveal melanoma. On indocyanine green angiography, the lesion is hypocyanescent with minimal late staining. OCT shows a characteristic "lumpy-bumpy" contour. Other features include choriocapillaris compression and subretinal fluid.
- The diagnosis is clinical. However, in cases where the features are atypical, fine-needle aspiration biopsy is useful.

- The management of uveal metastasis includes external beam radiotherapy, plaque radiotherapy, systemic chemotherapy, systemic targeted medications, and photodynamic therapy.

Acknowledgment

The authors would like to thank Kevin Card, BS, Ocular Oncology Service, Wills Eye Hospital for helping with the illustrations.

CHAPTER 56

Choroid Hemangioma Circumscribed

Nicholas E. Kalafatis ■ Saaquib Bakhsh ■ Denis Jusufbegovic

Decreased Visual Acuity in a 53-Year-Old Male

HISTORY OF PRESENT ILLNESS

A 53-year-old male presented to his optometrist for a gradual decline in visual acuity in the left eye (OS) of unclear duration. He was referred to a general ophthalmologist for further evaluation, who confirmed central vision and nonspecific visual field loss OS. On dilated fundus examination, no other ocular abnormalities were recognized, and the patient was diagnosed with a possible optic neuropathy. He was subsequently evaluated by a neuroophthalmologist who ruled out this diagnosis but discovered cystoid macular edema (CME) on optical coherence tomography (OCT) and referred him to our retina clinic for evaluation.

Exam

	OD	OS
Visual acuity	20/20	20/400
IOP (mm Hg)	15	14
Sclera/conjunctiva	White and quiet	White and quiet
Cornea	Clear	Clear
AC	Deep and quiet	Deep and quiet
Iris	Round, no NVI	Round, no NVI
Lens	Clear	Clear
Anterior vitreous	Clear	Clear
Retina/optic nerve	Optic nerve normal, retina flat, macula intact	8 mm × 7 mm × 2.8 mm pinkish-orange, amelanotic mass near superior arcade with SRF extending into the macula

AC, Anterior chamber; *IOP*, intraocular pressure; *NVI*, neovascularization of the iris; *SRF*, subretinal fluid.

QUESTIONS TO ASK

- Have you ever had previous episodes of blurred vision in the affected eye?
- Have you ever had fundus photographs taken?
- Do you have a history of Sturge-Weber syndrome?
- Do you have a history of cancer?

No financial interest associated with the manuscript. No funding supports.

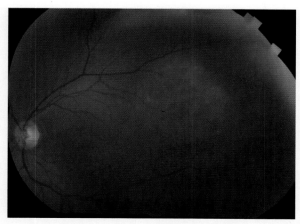

Fig. 56.1 Fundus photograph of the left eye depicting an 8 mm × 7 mm, raised, red-orange choroidal mass and changes consistent with subretinal fluid (SRF) in the macula.

The patient never had prior episodes of blurry vision. He never had fundus photographs taken. His past medical and ocular history was unremarkable, and family history was only notable for age-related macular degeneration in his mother. There is no personal or family history of cancer or Sturge-Weber syndrome.

ASSESSMENT

- Pinkish-orange, amelanotic choroidal mass, OS
- Subretinal fluid (SRF) and CME involving fovea

DIFFERENTIAL DIAGNOSIS

- Choroidal hemangioma circumscribed (CHC)
- Choroidal metastasis
- Amelanotic choroidal melanoma
- Choroidal lymphoma
- Posterior scleritis

WORKING DIAGNOSIS

- CHC, OS

INVESTIGATION AND TESTING

- Fundus photographs captured the well-circumscribed pinkish-orange choroidal mass (Fig. 56.1). The mass somewhat blends into the normal surrounding fundus on dilated fundus examination and can easily be overlooked by inexperienced observers.
- Fluorescein angiography (FA) and indocyanine green angiography (ICGA) demonstrated early prearterial hyperfluorescence and late staining of the mass on FA and early hyperfluoresence followed by characteristic hypofluorescence (described as washout) on the late stages of the ICG angiogram (Fig. 56.2).

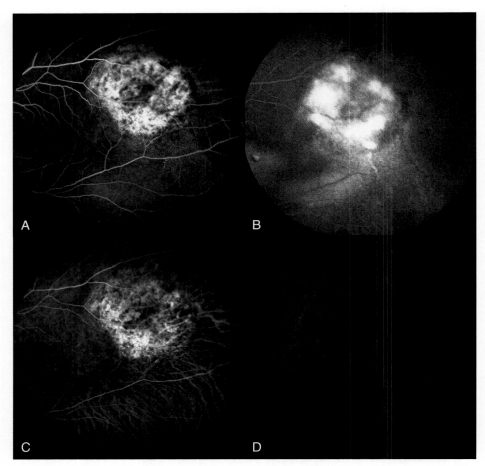

Fig. 56.2 Fluorescein angiography of the left eye demonstrating (A) early hyperfluorescence of the mass with (B) staining in later stages. (C) Indocyanine green angiography (ICGA) showing early hyperfluorescence of the mass (D) with washout in later stages.

- OCT showed subretinal and intraretinal fluid involving the macula and evidence of the dome-shaped mass arising in the choroid with no compression of the choriocapillaris (Fig. 56.3).
- B-scan ultrasonography revealed a 2.8-mm echodense mass with high internal reflectivity on A-scan (Fig. 56.4).

MANAGEMENT

- The patient underwent bevacizumab injection OS followed by photodynamic therapy (PDT) 2 weeks later with full-dose (6 mg/m²) verteporfin, full fluence (50 J/cm²), and double duration (83 sec × 2).

FOLLOW-UP

- There was a complete resolution of SRF, and tumor thickness was reduced to 1.5 mm. The patient's visual acuity improved to 20/100. OCT showed significant subfoveal outer retinal disruption, most likely related to the presence of chronic SRF before therapy.

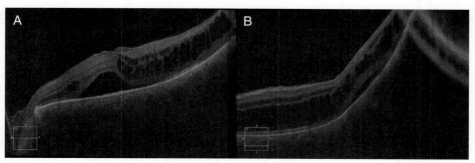

Fig. 56.3 (A) Optical coherence tomography (OCT) revealing intraretinal fluid and evidence of ellipsoid zone deterioration in the fovea. (B) Raster over the lesion confirming the dome-shaped mass arises in the choroid.

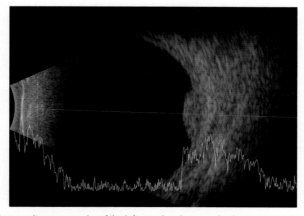

Fig. 56.4 A- and B-scan ultrasonography of the left eye showing an echodense mass arising from the choroid.

KEY POINTS

- CHC is a sporadic, benign, vascular tumor that often presents with visual acuity changes in adults.
- This tumor must be differentiated from more aggressive neoplasms, including uveal melanoma and uveal metastases. A metastatic carcinoid tumor may closely mimic choroidal hemangioma given its orange appearance. Using multimodal imaging, including A- and B-scan ultrasonography, fluorescein and ICG angiography, and OCT, CHC can be distinguished from other lesions.
- Pinkish-orange appearance of the mass with subtle elevation may camouflage with the normal surrounding fundus and go unrecognized during a cursory examination.
- When symptomatic, treatment is indicated. Visual changes are typically caused by secondary SRF and CME, and less frequently by subretinal fibrosis, retinoschisis, or retinal pigment epithelium (RPE) changes.
- These tumors respond well to laser photocoagulation, PDT, transpupillary thermotherapy (TTT), external beam radiotherapy, and plaque brachytherapy; however, in very rare cases enucleation may be required in the setting of neovascular glaucoma.
- Currently, PDT is a preferred therapeutic option for CHC, and radiotherapy is reserved for symptomatic cases resistant to PDT. The majority of treated patients experience improvement in visual acuity.

CHAPTER 57

Choroid Hemangioma Diffuse

Mona Camacci ■ Vikas Khetan

Decreased Visual Acuity in an 11-Year-Old Child

HISTORY OF PRESENT ILLNESS

An 11-year-old female presents with changes in vision in the left eye for 2 months. She feels as though she has had difficulty focusing at school. Past ocular history includes amblyopia in the left eye for which she had undergone treatment when younger. Her mother reports that the child has had a large facial birthmark since birth.

Exam

	OD	OS
Visual acuity	20/20	20/100
IOP (mm Hg)	20	24
Sclera/conjunctiva	White and quiet	White and quiet
Cornea	Clear	Clear
AC	Deep and quiet	Deep and quiet
Iris	Normal shape, size, and morphology	Normal shape, size, and morphology
Lens	Normal cortex, nuclear, and anterior and posterior capsule	Normal cortex, nuclear, and anterior and posterior capsule
	Clear	Clear
Anterior vitreous	Clear	Clear
Retina/optic nerve	Normal optic nerve with cup-to-disc ratio of 0.3	Normal optic nerve with cup-to-disc ratio of 0.3
	Posterior and peripheral retina normal	Vessels and macula normal
		Superior and temporal retinal elevation

AC, Anterior chamber; *IOP*, intraocular pressure.

QUESTIONS TO ASK

- Are there any previous neurological findings, such as seizures?
- Is there any history of neurological imaging?
- Does the child have any other relevant medical history?

The patient was diagnosed with a port-wine stain in the V1 distribution of the trigeminal nerve as a child. There is no history of seizures, and an MRI previously performed did not show any leptomeningeal enhancement. There is no history of cancer in the family. Parents deny any other significant medical history.

No financial interest associated with the manuscript. No funding supports.

ASSESSMENT

- Retinal elevation with thickening of the choroid, OS, suggestive of diffuse choroidal hemangioma

DIFFERENTIAL DIAGNOSIS

- Diffuse choroidal hemangioma
- Amelanotic melanoma
- Choroidal osteoma
- Choroidal metastasis

WORKING DIAGNOSIS

- Diffuse choroidal hemangioma, OS, secondary to Sturge-Weber syndrome

INVESTIGATION AND TESTING

- Retinal imaging showed diffuse choroidal hemangioma with discoloration of the retina diffusely (Figs. 57.1 and 57.2).
- B-scan ultrasound of OS showed choroidal thickening (Fig. 57.3).

MANAGEMENT

- The patient underwent photodynamic therapy OS.
- Symptoms improved with the photodynamic therapy.

FOLLOW-UP

- The patient presented 3 years later with vision loss from 20/50 to 20/200 OS with new subretinal fluid (SRF) in areas previously treated with photodynamic therapy (Fig. 57.4).
- The patient underwent external beam radiation.

KEY POINTS

- Diffuse choroidal hemangiomas typically occur in children and are mostly associated with Sturge-Weber syndrome. Roughly 40% of patients with Sturge-Weber syndrome will have choroidal hemangioma.

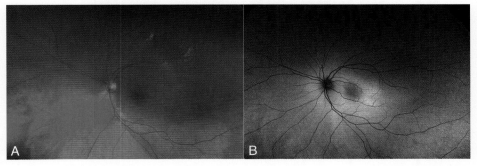

Fig. 57.1 (A) Optos photographs and (B) autofluorescence of the left eye at initial presentation showing a diffuse choroidal hemangioma with a small amount of subretinal fluid (SRF) superiorly and temporally.

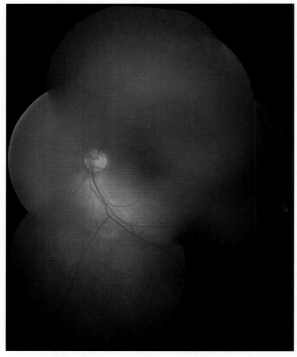

Fig. 57.2 Fundus photographs showing a diffuse choroidal hemangioma with a small amount of subretinal fluid (SRF) superiorly and temporally.

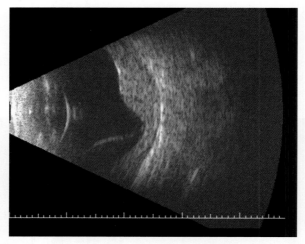

Fig. 57.3 B-scan ultrasound showing choroidal thickening and retinal elevation.

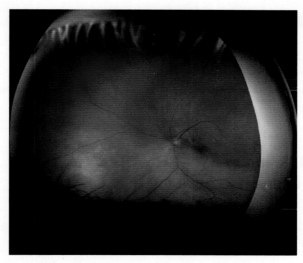

Fig. 57.4 Optos fundus photograph of left eye at follow-up presentation showing a diffuse choroidal heman-gioma with new infratemporal exudative retinal detachment.

■ The management of diffuse choroidal hemangioma is dependent on the extent of the tumor and presence of secondary retinal detachment. If the tumor has minimal elevation without significant SRF, patients can be observed and the prognosis is good. For thicker tumors or when SRF is present, treatment can include oral propranolol, photodynamic therapy, plaque radiotherapy, and external beam radiation with a more guarded prognosis.

CHAPTER 58

Choroid Osteoma

Vicktoria Vishnevskia-Dai ■ Ofira Zloto

Decreased Vision in a 29-Year-Old Male

HISTORY OF PRESENT ILLNESS

A previously healthy 29-year-old male presented with left eye decreased visual acuity.

Exam

	OD	OS
Visual acuity	20/20	20/100, ph 20/40
IOP (mm Hg)	13	14
Sclera/conjunctiva	White and quiet	White and quiet
Cornea	Clear	Clear
AC	Deep and quiet	Deep and quiet
Iris	Unremarkable, brown iris, no NVI	Unremarkable, brown iris, no NVI
Pupil	Round reactive	Round reactive, no RAPD
Lens	Clear	Clear
Anterior vitreous	Clear	Clear
Retina/optic nerve	Normal optic nerve, posterior and peripheral retina	Normal optic nerve, white flat macular lesion noted adjacent to the disc occupying all the macula between the arcades
		Normal peripheral retina (Fig. 58.1)

AC, Anterior chamber; *IOP,* intraocular pressure; *NVI,* neovascularization of the iris; *ph,* pinhole; *RAPD,* relative afferent pupillary defect.

QUESTIONS TO ASK

- Are you healthy?
- Do you have any history of weight loss, night sweating, or night fever?
- Do you smoke?
- Is there any history of cancer in the family?

The patient is a healthy nonsmoking man. He has never complained of weight loss, night sweating, or night fever. There is no history of cancer in the family.

No financial interest associated with the manuscript. No funding supports.

ASSESSMENT

■ Macular choroidal lesion with subretinal fluid (SRF), OS

DIFFERENTIAL DIAGNOSIS

■ Choroidal osteoma
■ Choroidal metastasis
■ Choroidal hemangioma
■ Amelanotic choroidal melanoma
■ Choroidal lymphoma
■ Choroidal granuloma
■ Choroiditis: tuberculosis, syphilis
■ Cytomegalovirus retinitis
■ Scleral choroidal calcifications

WORKING DIAGNOSIS

■ Choroidal osteoma

INVESTIGATION AND TESTING

■ Fundus photography (Fig. 58.1) showed a yellowish-white lesion superotemporal to the optic nerve with surrounding fluid.
■ B-scan ultrasound of the left eye showed a hyperreflective choroidal mass with dark acoustic shadowing, and an A-scan showed a high-intensity echo spike. (Fig. 58.2).
■ Optical coherence tomography (OCT) showed subfoveal fluid (Fig. 58.3).
■ Fluorescein angiography showed early patchy choroidal hyperfluorescence with late diffuse choroidal staining without foveolar involvement and without choroidal neovascular membrane (Fig. 58.4).

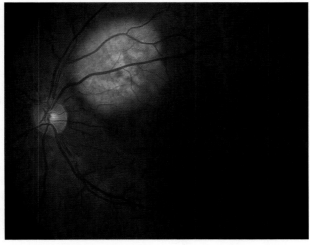

Fig. 58.1 Extrafoveal choroidal osteoma with subretinal fluid.

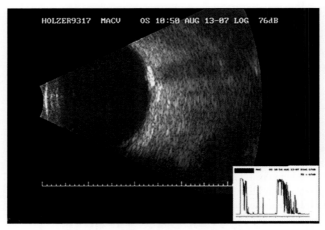

Fig. 58.2 B-scan ultrasound depicting hyperreflective choroidal mass with dark acoustic shadowing. A-scan ultrasound shows a high-intensity echo spike.

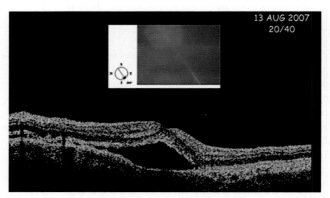

Fig. 58.3 Spectral-domain optical coherence tomography depicting subfoveal subretinal fluid without choroidal neovascularization (CNV).

MANAGEMENT

- The patient underwent photodynamic therapy (PDT) to the left eye with the intention to prevent tumor growth into the macula. Yet massive SRF formation led to a temporary visual decrease. Spontaneous resolution of the fluid was noted 2 months post-PDT with full vision recovery.

FOLLOW-UP

- Tumor growth was noted (Fig. 58.5) 1 year post-PDT, and a choroidal neovascularization with SRF was depicted on fluorescein angiography (Fig. 58.6) and OCT (Fig. 58.7).
- The patient required several round of anti-VEGF injections. With time, the lesion showed additional growth and atrophy of the overlying retina that led to irreversible decreased visual acuity.
- The visual acuity continued to decrease, and a central inferior scotoma developed in the left eye. The patient's final visual acuity was 20/400 with a stable osteoma.

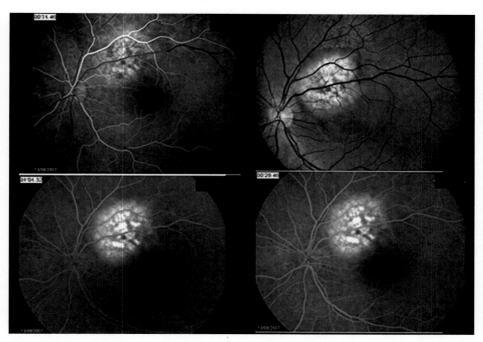

Fig. 58.4 Fluorescein angiography depicting early patchy choroidal hyperfluorescence with late diffuse choroidal staining without foveolar involvement and without choroidal neovascularization (CNV).

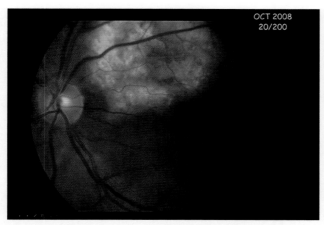

Fig. 58.5 Color fundus photography 1 year post–photodynamic therapy depicting growth of the choroidal osteoma with a pink central area suspicious of choroidal neovascularization.

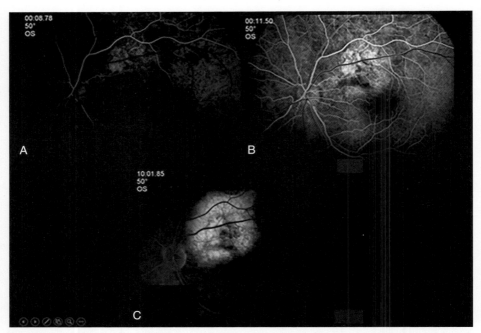

Fig. 58.6 Fluorescein angiography depicting early patchy choroidal hyperfluorescence with late diffuse choroidal staining and central hyperfluorescence compatible with choroidal neovascularization (CNV). (A) Early arterial phase (B) Laminar flow (C) Late phase.

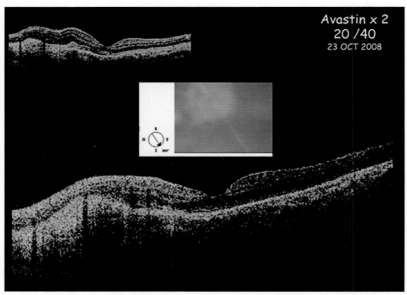

Fig. 58.7 Spectral domain optical coherence tomography depicting regression of the hyperintense areas compatible with inactive choroidal neovascularization (CNV).

KEY POINTS

- Choroidal osteoma is a rare benign tumor composed of mature bone replacing the full thickness of the choroid.
- It usually presents as an asymptomatic, unilateral (in 79% of eyes), orange-yellow plaque with clumping of brown, black, or gray pigment. Tumor growth is observed in 51%, choroidal neovascularization (CNV) in 31% over 10 years, and CNV in 46% after 20 years of follow-up.
- The tumor can undergo a process of spontaneous decalcification in 46% of the tumors by 10 years. Yet decalcification also can be induced by laser photocoagulation or PDT.
- SRF with or without choroidal neovascular membranes (CNVM) are the main complications leading to visual disturbances.

CHAPTER 59

Choroid Primary Lymphoma

Nathalie Cassoux ■ Denis Malaise ■ Alexandre Matet

A 56-Year-Old Female Was Referred for Choroidal Infiltration of the Right Eye

HISTORY OF PRESENT ILLNESS

A 56-year-old female was referred for a choroidal infiltration of the right eye. She complained of visual loss of the right eye over several months without any pain. Patient had no significant medical history.

Exam

	OD	OS
Visual acuity	20/100	20/20
IOP (mm Hg)	15	16
Sclera/conjunctiva	White and quiet	White and quiet
Cornea	Clear	Clear
AC	Deep and quiet	Deep and quiet
Iris	Unremarkable	Unremarkable
Lens	Clear	Clear
Anterior vitreous	Clear and quiet	Clear and quiet
Retina/optic nerve	Yellowish thick choroid with choroidal folds, areas of exudative retinal detachment, papilledema	Normal

AC, Anterior chamber; *IOP,* intraocular pressure.

QUESTIONS TO ASK

■ Do you have any past medical history of cancer?
■ Do you experience pain in your right eye?

There is no history of cancer and no significant past medical history. The patient has never complained of pain or redness in the right eye.

ASSESSMENT

■ Choroidal infiltration, OD (Fig. 59.1)

No financial interest associated with the manuscript. No funding supports.

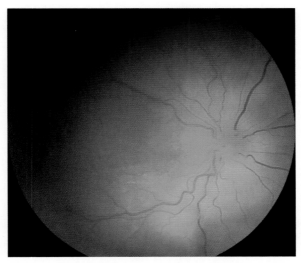

Fig. 59.1 Fundus photography of the right eye shows a yellowish infiltration of the choroid, choroidal folds and papilledema.

DIFFERENTIAL DIAGNOSIS

- Choroidal metastasis
- Achromic infiltrative choroidal melanoma
- Choroidal lymphoma, primitive or secondary
- Diffuse choroidal hemangioma
- Posterior/anterior scleritis
- Uveitis, birdshot uveitis, white dot syndrome

SYSTEMIC WORKUP

- Chest/abdominal CT scan
- Positron emission tomography (PET) scan

No primitive cancer or systemic lymphoma was found that could have metastasized to the choroid.

WORKING DIAGNOSIS

- Primary choroidal MALT lymphoma

INVESTIGATION AND TESTING

- Fluorescein angiography showed hyperfluorescent areas associated with hypofluorescent lesions and a peripapillary exudative detachment (Fig. 59.2).
- With optical coherence tomography (OCT), choroid looked irregular and thick and associated with localized exudative retinal detachment.
- Ultrasound ocular echography showed a hypoechogenic infiltration at the choroid level and a thickening of the sclera and episclera (Fig. 59.3).

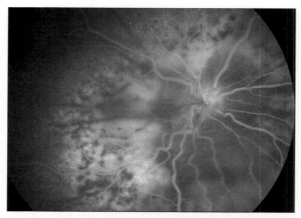

Fig. 59.2 Fluorescein angiography shows hypofluorescent areas of choroidal infiltration associated with exudative retinal detachment and hyperfluorescent lesions with pinpoints and papilledema.

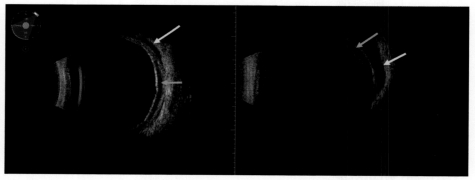

Fig. 59.3 On ultrasonography, choroidal *(orange arrows)* and scleral and episcleral infiltration *(yellow arrows)* are hypoechogenic, achieving a double black-coat appearance.

- Orbital MRI disclosed a deformation of the eyeball, a thickening of the choroid enhanced by gadolinium, and abnormal tissue in the episcleral position (Fig. 59.4).

MANAGEMENT

- Based on MRI and ocular ultrasound findings, an ab externo biopsy was organized.
- Exploration of the superotemporal quadrant disclosed an abnormal pinkish tissue along the sclera that was biopsied (Fig. 59.5).
- Histology revealed an infiltration composed of small lymphocytes, positive for CD20, CD79a, and BCL2 and organized around small germinative centers. Tumor cells produced monoclonal IgG *kappa*.
- The final diagnosis was primary choroidal MALT lymphoma.
- Hematologic systemic workup did not find any other location of MALT lymphoma.
- Treatment consisted of low-dose external beam radiotherapy, with 24 Gy administered in 12 fractions.

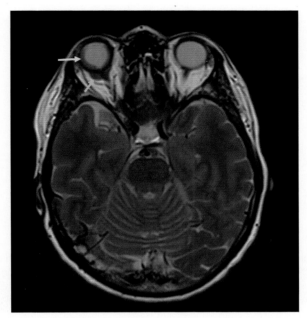

Fig. 59.4 T2-weighted ocular MRI shows an infiltration of the choroid *(yellow arrow)* and the episclera *(orange arrow)* when the sclera remains black.

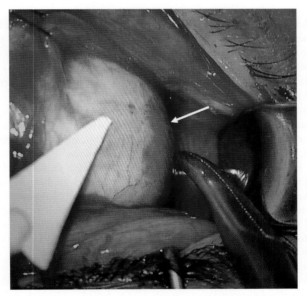

Fig. 59.5 Ab externo per operative biopsy guided by ultrasound echography. The pink tumor infiltration is located close to the vortex vein *(white arrow)*.

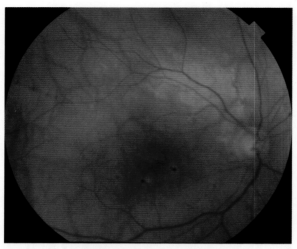

Fig. 59.6 Fundus photography after low-dose external beam radiotherapy. Tumoral infiltration has completely regressed. Scattered retinal pigmented epithelium alterations remain visible.

FOLLOW-UP

- Infiltration regressed completely, leaving scars on the fundus. Patient maintained good visual acuity of 20/25 during 6 years of follow-up without any relapse (Fig. 59.6).

KEY POINTS

- Primary choroidal MALT lymphoma may present various and nonspecific features. Involvement of the uvea can be uni- or bilateral. This condition can involve the anterior uvea, the choroid, or both. Owing to its insidious onset and its ability to simulate other conditions, the diagnosis is commonly delayed.
- A better knowledge of suggestive imaging findings (ocular ultrasonography and MRI) would also facilitate early diagnosis.
- The most suggestive imaging is ocular ultrasonography showing hypoechogenic thick choroid associated with episcleral hypoechogenic mass. MRI of the orbit is also useful, showing a contrast-enhanced thick choroid, eyeball deformation, and contrast-enhanced episcleral infiltration, localized or diffuse, around the optic nerve head.
- Histologic evidence remains mandatory for the diagnosis of choroidal MALT lymphoma. The first option consists of performing superficial biopsy on the most accessible localization. Conjunctival or Tenon capsule biopsy is a safe and minimally invasive technique and must be considered as a first-line procedure. These ab externo biopsies are most often conclusive. Superficial and deep episcleral or scleral biopsies are also performed and may constitute an alternative when no superficial site is available. In some rare cases, ab interno choroidal biopsy may be necessary.
- Hematologic workup is necessary to exclude any other mucosal location.
- Management consists of low-dose external beam radiotherapy alone or combined with chemotherapy or chemotherapy alone (by anti-CD20 drugs).
- Usually, this disease carries a very good prognosis.

CHAPTER 60

Retina Vasoproliferative Tumor

Joseph Luvisi ■ Emil Anthony Say

Decreased Vision and Floaters in a 23-Year-Old Female

HISTORY OF PRESENT ILLNESS

A 23-year-old female presented for decreased vision with floaters in the right eye (OD) for more than 6 months and floaters in the left eye (OS) for 1 month.

Exam

	OD	OS
Visual acuity	20/150	20/30
IOP (mmHg)	18	16
Sclera/conjunctiva	White and quiet	White and quiet
Cornea	Clear	Clear
AC	Deep and quiet	Deep and quiet
Iris	Round	Round
Lens	1+ NS	Clear
Anterior vitreous	Normal for age	Normal for age
Optic Nerve	Pink and sharp	Pink and sharp
Macula	Inferior exudation	Blunted reflex
Vessels	Dilated and tortuous mostly inferiorly	Dilated and tortuous mostly inferiorly and close to tumor
Periphery	Inferior subretinal lipid exudation and SRF associated with an inferotemporal yellowish-pink tumor peripherally (Fig. 60.1A)	Inferotemporal peripheral yellowish-pink tumor with surrounding lipid exudation (Fig. 60.1B)

AC, Anterior chamber; *IOP,* intraocular pressure; *NS,* nuclear sclerosis; *SRF,* subretinal fluid.

QUESTIONS TO ASK

- Is this the first time you have had floaters and decreased vision?
- Do you have any significant ocular, medical, or birth history?
- Do you have any family history of hereditary diseases or tumors?

The patient reports multiple episodes of decreased vision and floaters in both eyes (OU) during childhood from having pars planitis and previously received treatment with steroids to control the inflammation. She was born term with normal birth weight and had no prior history of eye disease apart from pars planitis. She has no known family history of hereditary diseases (both ocular and extraocular), malignancy, or tumors.

No financial interest associated with the manuscript. No funding supports.

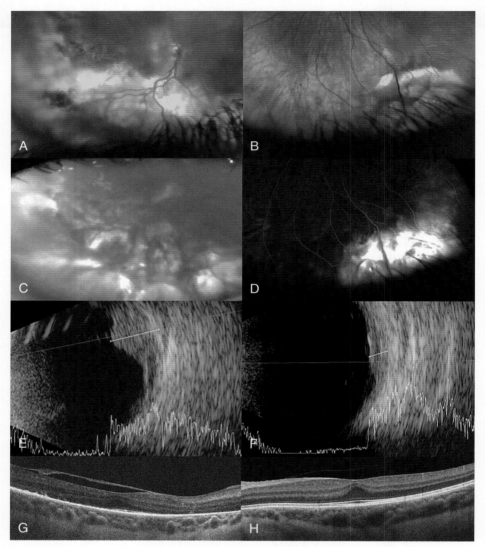

Fig. 60.1   (A) A 23-year-old female with prior history of pars planitis developed bilateral secondary vasoproliferative tumors seen as yellowish-pink tumors in the inferotemporal periphery with adjacent subretinal fluid
(SRF) and lipid exudation worse in the right eye (OD) than (B) the left (OS). Fluorescein angiography shows late
leakage, most emanating from the inferotemporal tumors, which also appear worse in (C) the OD than (D) the
OS. (E) Ultrasonography shows dome-shaped echodense tumors with adjacent SRF that measures 7.5 mm
in thickness OD and (F) 2.7 mm OS. (G) Horizontal optical coherence tomography (OCT) across the fovea
shows bilateral epiretinal membrane formation with more prominent macular traction and loss of ellipsoid
temporally OD (H) that was not appreciated OS.

ASSESSMENT

- Unifocal inferotemporal retinal tumors with feeder vessels associated with subretinal fluid (SRF) and lipid exudation OU in the setting of prior history of pars planitis OU

DIFFERENTIAL DIAGNOSIS

- Retinal vasoproliferative tumor
- Retinal capillary hemangioma
- Retinal cavernous hemangioma
- Choroidal hemangioma
- Coats disease

WORKING DIAGNOSIS

- Secondary retinal vasoproliferative tumors associated with pars planitis OU

INVESTIGATION AND TESTING

- Fluorescein angiography shows ill-defined area of inferotemporal hyperfluorescence associated with late leakage involving the adjacent retina OD (Fig. 60.1C), more than OS (Fig. 60.1D).
- Ultrasonography shows bilateral dome-shaped echodense mass measuring 7.5 mm OD (Fig. 60.1E) and 2.3 mm OS (Fig. 60.1F) with adjacent SRF OU.
- Optical coherence tomography (OCT) shows epiretinal membrane OU with macular traction and loss of ellipsoid OD likely from chronic exudation or macular edema (Fig. 60.1G–H).

MANAGEMENT

- Patient underwent plaque radiotherapy OD and cryotherapy OS.

FOLLOW-UP

- There was improvement in exudative retinal detachment and tumor regression OU (Fig. 60.2A–B).
- The patient's epiretinal membrane persisted OU but with improved macular traction OD (Fig. 60.2C–D). She subsequently developed cystoid macular edema (CME) OD 3–4 months after radiation treated with intravitreal anti–vascular endothelial growth factor (anti-VEGF) injection and intravitreal fluocinolone acetonide implant.
- During the 15-month follow-up, visual acuity was 20/80 OD and 20/30 OS without tumor recurrence, active exudation, or recurrent macular edema.

KEY POINTS

- Retinal vasoproliferative tumors are benign retinal vascular tumors that are usually solitary and typically located inferotemporal between the equator and ora serrata.
- They are primary (idiopathic) in 80%, while secondary retinal vasoproliferative tumors are most often associated with retinitis pigmentosa, pars planitis, and Coats disease.

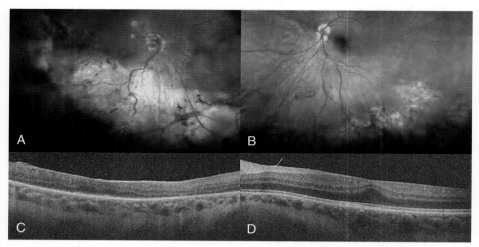

Fig. 60.2 Following plaque radiotherapy for the right eye (OD) and cryotherapy for the left (OS), tumor regression was noted in both eyes (OU) along with improvement in vision. (A) Fundus photographs at the patient's 15-month follow-up visit show inferior retinal pigment epithelium (RPE) atrophy despite resolution of subretinal fluid (SRF) and lipid exudation likely from chronic disease OD, (B) while the OS shows similar RPE atrophy. (C) Optical coherence tomography (OCT) OD shows release of macular traction with stable ellipsoid loss OD, and (D) OS shows stable epiretinal membrane (D).

- Tumors appear yellow-orange and may be associated with a dilated feeding artery and draining vein. In addition, adjacent intraretinal and subretinal exudation, SRF, and retinal pigment epithelium changes are common.
- Differentiating retinal vasoproliferative tumors from other vascular tumors and Coats disease can be done clinically but may sometimes require additional imaging.
  - Retinal capillary hemangiomas can be isolated or secondary to von Hippel-Lindau disease, with the latter association often leading to bilateral and multifocal tumors, as well as extraocular malignancy. Retinal capillary hemangiomas appear as well-circumscribed, orange-red tumors either in a juxtapapillary or peripheral location. Peripheral tumors will often have dilated and prominent feeder vessels, but those in both locations can be associated with lipid exudation and SRF.
  - Retinal cavernous hemangiomas appear as grapelike clusters of blood-filled aneurysmal lesions involving the inner retinal layers. They are often associated with adjacent epiretinal membranes but lack feeder vessels, exudation, or SRF.
  - Choroidal hemangiomas can be circumscribed or diffuse, with the latter usually associated with Sturge-Weber syndrome. They appear as pinkish-red tumors with either well-circumscribed (circumscribed) or ill-defined (diffuse) margins. Intraretinal and SRF overlying the tumor are frequent, but lipid exudation and feeder vessels are uncommon. Fluorescein angiography shows very early hyperfluorescence, whereas OCT localizes these tumors in the choroid with overlying retinal changes.
  - The distinguishing feature of Coats disease is peripheral retinal telangiectatic and aneurysmal changes that develop in association with more peripheral nonperfusion and are not typically seen with other retinal vascular tumors. Adjacent subretinal exudation and remote macular exudation are typical, and a distinct tumor is absent, although secondary vasoproliferative tumors in eyes with Coats disease can develop in rare instances. Advanced cases are associated with total exudative retinal detachment or neovascular glaucoma.

- Treatment options include observation, cryotherapy, thermal laser, photodynamic therapy, plaque radiotherapy, anti-VEGF injections, resection, and immunotherapy. Patients with small tumors are often asymptomatic and may be observed with little change to their vision; however, those with significant vision loss usually require treatment. Most tumors measuring 3.0 mm or less in thickness can be treated successfully with laser, cryotherapy, or photodynamic therapy, but those with greater thickness may require radiation or combination therapy with multiple modalities.
- Prognosis can vary. Vision loss associated with vasoproliferative tumors can be from macular edema, lipid exudation, vitreomacular traction, epiretinal membrane, exudative retinal detachment, and neovascular glaucoma.

CHAPTER 61

Retina Hemangioblastoma

Thomas A. DeCesare ■ Aparna Ramasubramanian

Left Inferior Retinal Mass in a 16-Year-Old Male With von Hippel-Lindau Syndrome

HISTORY OF PRESENT ILLNESS

A 16-year-old male with history of von Hippel-Lindau syndrome (VHL) was seen in the cancer predisposition clinic for routine surveillance. MRI brain/spine reveals a 2-mm-round contrast-enhancing mass in the left inferior globe abutting the retina. The patient was referred to the ophthalmology clinic for detailed evaluation.

Exam

	OD	OS
Visual acuity	Fix-and-follow	Fix-and-follow
IOP (mm Hg)	14	15
Sclera/conjunctiva	White and quiet	White and quiet
Cornea	Clear	Clear
AC	Deep and quiet	Deep and quiet
Iris	Brown iris, pupil round, no NVI	Brown iris, pupil round, no NVI
Lens	Clear	Clear
Anterior vitreous	Clear	Clear
Retina/optic nerve	Normal optic nerve and macula	Normal optic nerve and macula
	Small elevated red lesion in the superior retina (Fig. 61.1A)	Elevated hemorrhagic lesion in the inferior retina with dilated feeder vessel (Fig. 61.2A)

AC, Anterior chamber; *IOP,* intraocular pressure; *NVI,* neovascularization of the iris.

QUESTIONS TO ASK

- Have you observed any pain or vision changes?
- Are any other family members diagnosed with VHL?
- Do these family members have any previous diagnoses of neurologic or ocular tumors?
- Do you have any systemic features of VHL that include benign or malignant lesions elsewhere in the body?

Patient reports no changes in vision or pain in either eye. Family history is significant for father, two brothers, and one sister with VHL. Pertinent positives include father's VHL-related complications of two hemangioblastomas of the brain, each surgically resected, and ablation of one retinal hemangioblastoma. The patient has benign pancreatic cysts, autism, and developmental delay.

No financial interest associated with the manuscript. No funding supports.

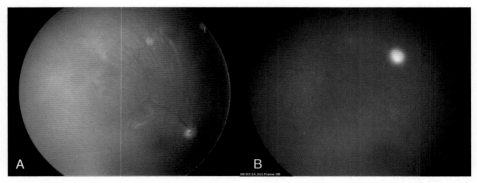

Fig. 61.1   (A) Retinal photo of right eye. (B) A superior hemangioblastoma with a possible small one just temporal to the larger one.

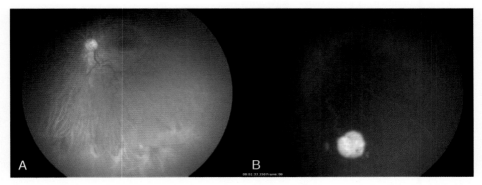

Fig. 61.2   (A) Retinal photo of the left eye. (B) An inferior hemangioblastoma with late leakage visualized using fluorescein angiography.

ASSESSMENT

- Bilateral elevated retinal lesion

DIFFERENTIAL DIAGNOSIS

- Retinal hemangioblastoma
- Retinoblastoma
- Astrocytoma

WORKING DIAGNOSIS

- Retinal hemangioblastoma, OU, secondary to VHL

INVESTIGATION AND TESTING

- Fluorescein angiography was done and showed a hyperfluorescent lesion in the superior retina, OD (Fig. 61.1B), and the inferior periphery OS (Fig. 61.2B).

MANAGEMENT

- Laser photocoagulation was performed on the right eye using a 532-nm laser and indirect ophthalmoscopy headpiece.
- Triple freeze-thaw cryotherapy of the left eye was performed.

FOLLOW-UP

- The patient has been monitored every 6 months with no new lesions and no recurrence of the hemangioblastoma.
- Ophthalmic screening of other family members with VHL was discussed.

KEY POINTS

- VHL syndrome is caused by a mutation to the VHL tumor suppressor gene on chromosome 3, leading to impaired ubiquitination and elimination of hypoxia-inducible factor 1a and subsequent cyst and tumor development.
- Hemangioblastomas are highly vascularized lesions of cells with hyperchromatic nuclei; they are common in patients with VHL.
- The most common locations of hemangioblastomas include the retina, cerebellum, brainstem, and spine.
- If left untreated, hemangioblastomas can cause vision loss and focal neurologic deficits. Annual dilated eye exams are warranted.
- The highest frequency of human gioblastomas is between ages 15 and 25.
- Central nervous system (CNS) hemangioblastomas are the most common cause of death in VHL patients.
- Patients with VHL should be screened biannually with CT/MRI of the brain and spine to detect hemangioblastomas beginning at age 11 years.

CHAPTER 62

Retina Astrocytoma

Kareem Sioufi ■ Andrew Stacey

Retinal Lesions in a 21-Year-Old Female

HISTORY OF PRESENT ILLNESS

A 21-year-old female presents as a referral from a local eye doctor for retinal lesions noted incidentally in both eyes during a routine examination. She denied any vision changes. The patient had no family history of ocular disease. She has no prior ocular history and has had no dilated eye exams.

Exam

	OD	OS
External	Small brown papules on cheeks and nose	Small brown papules on cheeks and nose
Visual acuity	20/20	20/20
IOP (mm Hg)	17	17
Sclera/conjunctiva	White and quiet	White and quiet
Cornea	Clear	Clear
AC	Deep and quiet	Deep and quiet
Iris	Normal	Normal
Lens	Clear	Clear
Vitreous	Normal	Normal
Retina/optic nerve	Multifocal inner retinal white lesions nasal to the nerve, multiple small lesions in the superior periphery	Multifocal inner retinal lesions, calcified mulberrylike lesion inferior to fovea

AC, Anterior chamber; *IOP,* intraocular pressure.

QUESTIONS TO ASK

- Do you have any skin lesions?
- Do you have a history of seizures?
- Is there a family history of ocular disease?

The patient did not have cutaneous depigmented macules (ash-leaf sign) and had never had seizures. She denied any other significant medical history. There was no family history of prior ocular disease.

No financial interest associated with the manuscript. No funding supports.

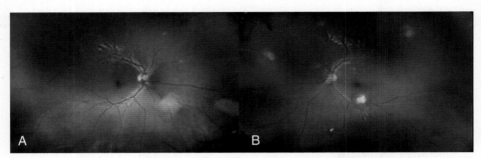

Fig. 62.1 (A) Ultrawide field imaging demonstrated multifocal inner retinal white lesions in the right eye. (B) The left eye showed similar lesions in the mid- and far periphery in addition to a mulberry-like calcified lesion inferior to the fovea and a smaller calcified lesion in the midperiphery.

ASSESSMENT

- Multiple pale retinal lesions, OU
- Calcified retinal lesion, OS

DIFFERENTIAL DIAGNOSIS

- Retinal astrocytic hamartoma (RAH)
- Retinal astrocytoma
- Retinoblastoma
- Myelinated nerve fiber layer

WORKING DIAGNOSIS

- Retinal astrocytic hamartoma, OU

INVESTIGATION AND TESTING

- Ultrawide field imaging demonstrated multifocal inner retinal white lesions, OD (Fig. 62.1A); the left eye (Fig. 62.1B) showed similar lesions in the mid- and far periphery in addition to a mulberry-like calcified lesion inferior to the fovea and a smaller calcified lesion in the midperiphery.
- Optical coherence tomography (OCT) OU demonstrated intact foveal contour. OCT OS through the lesion (Fig. 62.2) shows overlying vitreous condensation, increased thickness of retinal nerve fiber layer, intralesional cysts, and calcification.

MANAGEMENT

- Patient underwent brain MRI and was found to have multiple bilateral subependymal nodules lining lateral ventricles and adjacent to the foramen of Monro.
- Genetic testing was positive for a clinically significant alteration in the *TSC2* gene.
- The patient was referred to medical genetics and neurology for evaluation of a new diagnosis of tuberous sclerosis.

FOLLOW-UP

- The patient did not require any further ocular treatment and has remained stable on follow-up for more than 5 years.

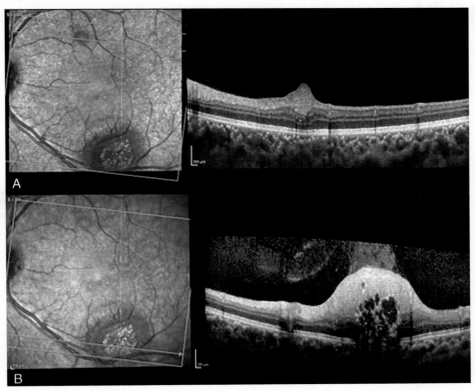

Fig. 62.2 (A) Optical coherence tomography (OCT) in the left eye through a small type 1 lesion superior to the fovea demonstrated increased retinal nerve fiber layer (RNFL) thickness. (B) OCT through a larger type 2 lesion inferior to the fovea showed overlying vitreous condensation, increased thickness RNFL with multiple intralesional optically empty spaces, and calcification.

KEY POINTS

- Retinal astrocytic hamartoma (RAH) is a glial tumor that can be found in isolation or in connection with tuberous sclerosis complex (TSC).
- It has been suggested that isolated retinal astrocytoma lesions not associated with TSC may demonstrate a more aggressive growth pattern while most RAHs associated with TSC lesions are circumscribed and demonstrate little effect to the surrounding retina.
- There are three morphological subtypes of RAH. Type 1 is relatively flat without calcifications. Type 2 is raised with calcification and a mulberry-like configuration. Type 3 is a transitional lesion with features of types 1 and 2.
- Treatment options include observation for inactive and small nonvisually significant tumors. When tumors are active, they may develop hemorrhage or retinal inflammation. In these situations, various treatments may be necessary, including laser (transpupillary thermotherapy [TTT] and photodynamic therapy [PDT] have both been used), radiation (external beam radiation or plaque radiotherapy), or medications including intravitreal injections of vascular endothelial growth factor (VEGF) inhibitors. In advanced astrocytoma tumors leading to neovascular glaucoma, enucleation may be required.
- The prognosis for RAH is generally good.

CHAPTER 63

Retina Congenital Hypertrophy of Retinal Pigment Epithelium

Margaret Reynolds ■ Jonathan Thomas

Left Retinal Lesions in a 5-Year-Old Child

HISTORY OF PRESENT ILLNESS

A healthy 5-year-old female presents with left retinal lesions after referral from a local physician to rule out familial adenomatous polyposis/Gardner syndrome. She has no visual complaints in either eye, and she has no history of ocular diseases.

Exam

	OD	OS
Visual acuity	20/20	20/20
IOP (mm Hg)	18	18
Sclera/conjunctiva	White and quiet	White and quiet
Cornea	Clear	Clear
AC	Deep and quiet	Deep and quiet
Iris	Round and reactive	Round and reactive
Lens	Clear	Clear
Anterior vitreous	Normal	Normal
Disc	Normal	Normal
C/D ratio	0.1	0.1
Macula	Normal	Normal
Vessels	Normal	Normal
Periphery	Normal	Normal, congenital hypertrophy of RPE appearance

AC, Anterior chamber; *IOP*, intraocular pressure; *RPE*, retinal pigment epithelium

QUESTIONS TO ASK

- Does the family have a history of cancer, particularly colon cancer?
- Does she have any other past medical history?
- Does she have any systemic symptoms (gastrointestinal, headaches, etc.)?

She has no family history of any types of cancer, including colon cancer. She has no other past medical history. Her systemic review of systems is negative.

No financial interest associated with the manuscript. No funding supports.

ASSESSMENT

- Grouped congenital hypertrophy of retinal pigment epithelium (RPE), OS

DIFFERENTIAL DIAGNOSIS

- Congenital hypertrophy of retinal pigment epithelium
- Choroidal nevus
- Choroidal melanoma
- Melanocytoma
- Focal pigmentation
- RPE hyperplasia
- Sunburst lesion in sickle cell

WORKING DIAGNOSIS

- Grouped congenital hypertrophy of RPE, OS

TESTING AND RESULTS

- Ultrawide-field imaging of the retinas was obtained, and round lesions in clusters were noted in OS (Figs. 63.1–63.4).

INVESTIGATION AND MANAGEMENT

- The patient did not require any active treatment to treat the lesions, and these lesions are not associated with Gardner syndrome.

FOLLOW-UP

- The patient was recommended to follow up in 1 year.

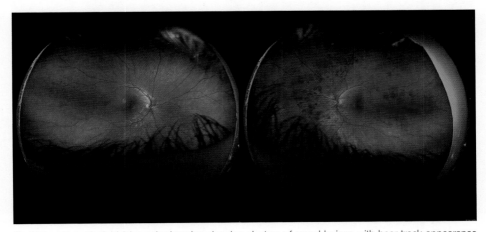

Fig. 63.1 Ultrawide-field false color imaging showing clusters of round lesions with bear-track appearance in the OS.

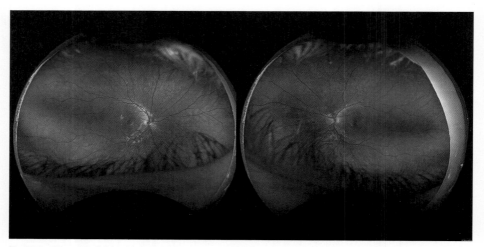

Fig. 63.2 Ultrawide-field red free imaging does not show clear differentiation of the lesions as it best visualizes lesions between neurosensory retina and retinal pigment epithelium.

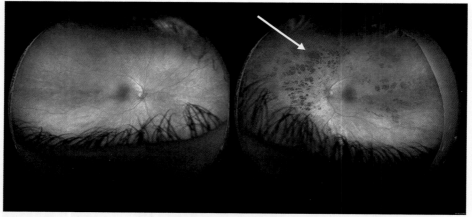

Fig. 63.3 Ultrawide-field green free imaging visualizes lesions between the retinal pigment epithelium and choroid. OS lesions are highlighted.

KEY POINTS

- Congenital hypertrophy of the retinal pigment epithelium (CHRPE) is an asymptomatic condition that presents with lesions in the retinal pigment epithelium layer.
- Depending on the characteristics of the lesions, the condition can be described as typical, grouped, or atypical congenital hypertrophy of the retinal pigment epithelium (CHRPE).
- Typical/solitary/unifocal CHRPE is characteristically single, flat, round, hyperpigmented retinal lesions. This lesion may be surrounded by a halo, which may enlarge over time.

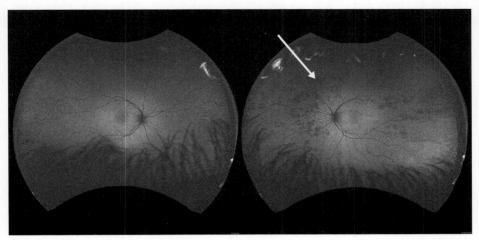

Fig. 63.4   The fundus autofluorescence shows hypoautofluorescence in the areas corresponding to the lesions.

- Atypical CHRPE, also called pigmented ocular fundus lesions (POFLs), are multiple, bilateral, oval, spindle, schistocyte, comma- or fishtail-shaped lesions irregularly distributed throughout the fundus. They represent retinal invasion and glial, capillary, and pigment epithelial proliferation and hypertrophy. These lesions are often bilateral (78% of patients).
- Despite confusion in the literature, only atypical CHRPE/POFL is associated with familial adenomatous polyposis; both typical and grouped CHRPE can proceed without concern or treatment.

CHAPTER **64**

Retinal Pigment Epithelium Adenoma/Adenocarcinoma

Bria George ■ Maura Di Nicola ■ Basil K. Williams, Jr.

Decreased Vision and Pigmented Lesion in a 52-Year-Old Female

HISTORY OF PRESENT ILLNESS

A 52-year-old White female presents with decreased vision and a referring diagnosis of pigmented lesion in the left eye. The patient had no prior ocular history of trauma. Medical history is significant for thyroid cancer.

Exam

	OD	OS
Visual acuity	20/20	20/80
IOP (mm Hg)	14	17
Sclera/conjunctiva	White and quiet	White and quiet
Cornea	Clear	Clear
AC	Deep and quiet	Deep and quiet
Iris	Unremarkable	Unremarkable
	Blue iris	Blue iris
Lens	Clear	Posterior chamber intraocular lens
Anterior vitreous	Clear	Clear
Retina/optic nerve	Normal optic nerve, posterior and peripheral retina	Normal optic nerve, posterior retina with cystoid macular edema and an epiretinal membrane
		Peripheral retina with an abruptly elevated mass arising from an area of combined hypertrophy of the RPE

AC, Anterior chamber; *IOP,* intraocular pressure; *RPE,* retinal pigment epithelium.

QUESTIONS TO ASK

- When was the last time you had a dilated exam?
- Have you experienced decreased or blurry vision?
- Do you have any history of ocular trauma?

No financial interest associated with the manuscript. No funding supports.

The patient had her last dilated exam several years prior. She had noticed decreased vision for the past 3–4 months and did not report any history of trauma.

ASSESSMENT

- Peripheral mass, OS
- Underlying combined hypertrophy of the retinal pigment epithelium (CHRPE)/chorioretinal scarring, OS
- Feeding artery and draining vessel, OS
- Subretinal exudation, OS

DIFFERENTIAL DIAGNOSIS

- Retinal pigment epithelium (RPE) adenoma/adenocarcinoma
- Choroidal melanoma
- Congenital hypertrophy of the RPE
- Hyperplasia of the RPE

WORKING DIAGNOSIS

- RPE adenoma/adenocarcinoma, OS

INVESTIGATION AND TESTING

- Fundus photography confirmed the presence of a peripheral elevated pigmented lesion with underlying CHRPE and surrounding exudation (Fig. 64.1A).
- B-scan ultrasound of OS showed a dense dome-shaped lesion of 2.5 mm in thickness. Vitreous debris arising from the lesion was also noted (Fig. 64.1B).
- A-scan ultrasound of the lesion demonstrated medium internal reflectivity.
- Fluorescein angiography revealed a mildly hyperfluorescent lesion in the early phase with midphase hyperfluorescence and late leakage (Fig. 64.1C–D).
- Optical coherence tomography (OCT) imaging of the peripheral lesion demonstrated an abruptly elevated lesion with high optical density, retinal invasion, a derby hat configuration, and posterior shadowing (Fig. 64.2A). OCT of the macula showed intraretinal and subretinal fluid (SRF) with an overlying epiretinal membrane (Fig. 64.2B).

MANAGEMENT

- A subtenon injection of triamcinolone acetonide was administered without significant improvement in the intraretinal fluid or SRF.
- The lesion continued to grow in basal dimensions, and photodynamic therapy was performed.

FOLLOW-UP

- The lesion did not show any additional growth, but the patient experienced progressive decreased vision to 20/150 over the following 4 years secondary to persistent edema.
- No additional treatment was performed due to patient preference.

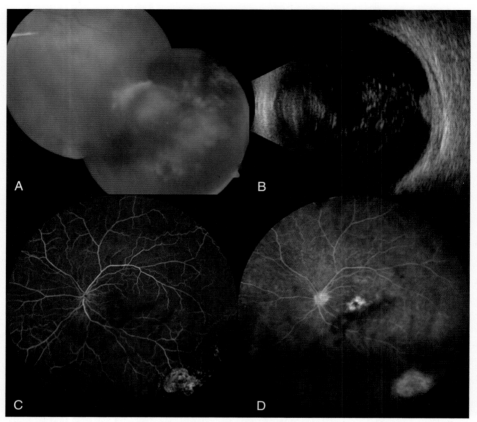

Fig. 64.1 (A) Fundus photography of the left eye demonstrating an elevated pigmented lesion arising from CHRPE with surrounding exudation. (B) B-scan ultrasonography shows a dense mass with abrupt elevation. (C) On fluorescein angiography, the mass appears mildly hyperfluorescent in the early phase (D) with late leakage.

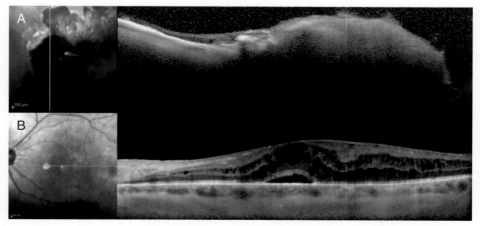

Fig. 64.2 (A) Optical coherence tomography (OCT) through the mass demonstrates an abruptly elevated lesion with high optical density and posterior shadowing. (B) OCT of the macula demonstrates intraretinal and subretinal fluid with an overlying epiretinal membrane.

KEY POINTS

- RPE adenoma/adenocarcinoma is commonly misdiagnosed as choroidal melanoma, occasionally resulting in avoidable enucleation.
- RPE adenoma/adenocarcinoma has clinical and imaging characteristics that help distinguish it from choroidal melanoma at presentation, including abrupt elevation, lipid exudation, presence of a feeding artery and/or draining vein, and underlying congenital hypertrophy of the RPE.
- Primary management is often observation, but a rapidly enlarging lesion or one causing vision-threatening complications may warrant treatment.
- Intravitreal injections of antivascular endothelial growth factor or steroids may reduce the exudative effects of this tumor but do not treat the underlying lesion.
- Other treatment options include photodynamic therapy, transpupillary thermotherapy, cryotherapy, plaque brachytherapy, and endo- or exoresection, but no specific treatment is universally successful.

CHAPTER 65

Primary Vitreoretinal Lymphoma

Janelle Marie Fassbender Adeniran

Chronic Floaters and Decreased Visual Acuity in a 69-Year-Old Female

HISTORY OF PRESENT ILLNESS

A 69-year-old female presents with chronic floaters and gradual worsening vision in both eyes. She has a history of uveitis and was referred for a second opinion. She is presently taking oral prednisone and using topical prednisolone acetate. She states that her vision gets worse when she does not take her pills.

Exam

	OD	OS
Visual acuity	20/60	20/100
IOP (mm Hg)	20	18
Sclera/conjunctiva	White and quiet	White and quiet
Cornea	Clear	Clear
AC	Absent cell and flare	Absent cell and flare
Iris	Unremarkable	Unremarkable
Lens	1+ NS	1+ NS
Anterior vitreous	3+ cells	1+ cells
Retina/optic nerve	3+ vitritis, poor view to optic nerve, pigmented chorioretinal lesion inferior to optic nerve	1+ vitritis, optic nerve pink and without edema, yellowish irregular retinal lesions within central macula and poorly defined lesions in the nasal periphery

AC, Anterior chamber; *IOP,* intraocular pressure; *NS,* nuclear sclerosis.

QUESTIONS TO ASK

- Do you have any known personal or familial autoimmune disease?
- Do you have any personal or family history of cancer?
- Do you have any history of immunosuppression?

The patient had a prophylactic mastectomy in 1992 and underwent a craniotomy in 2018 for a brain lesion that was initially thought to be lymphoma, but a pathology second opinion stated it was probable a benign lesion. She had been on 40 mg of prednisone for 4 months but refused to taper because her vision would worsen.

No financial interest associated with the manuscript. No funding supports.

ASSESSMENT

- Dense vitritis, OD
- Milder vitritis with small, multifocal, retinal infiltrates, OS

DIFFERENTIAL DIAGNOSIS

- Vitreoretinal lymphoma (VRL)
- Intermediate uveitis with choroidal granulomas
- Choroidal metastasis

WORKING DIAGNOSIS

- Vitreoretinal lymphoma, OU

INVESTIGATION AND TESTING

- Fundus color and autofluorescence photography (Fig. 65.1).
- OCT (Fig. 65.2).

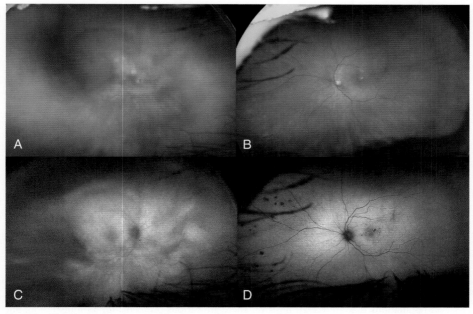

Fig. 65.1 (A) Color fundus photo and fundus autofluorescence of the right eye demonstrating significant vitritis with poorly viewed optic disc features and chorioretinal lesion inferior to the disc. (B) Color fundus photo of the left eye shows the yellowish, irregular retinal lesions within the central macula as well as poorly defined lesions in the nasal periphery and are more clearly demonstrated due to less vitritis. (C) Corresponding fundus autofluorescence is significantly blocked due to vitritis of the right eye (D) but reveals hypoautofluorescent lesions in the left eye.

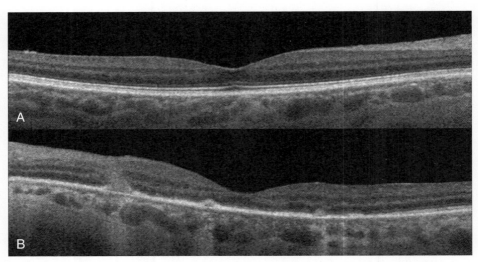

Fig. 65.2 (A) Optical coherence tomography after vitrectomy in the right eye reveals a mild epiretinal membrane with a normal retinal structure and (B) multifocal hyperreflective lesions in the left eye affecting all retinal layers including infiltration of the choroid.

MANAGEMENT

- Patient underwent diagnostic vitrectomy of OD, which confirmed a diagnosis of B-cell lymphoma.
- Additional systemic testing included restaging with whole body CT and PET; and MRI brain, which revealed no new findings compared to prior imaging.
- She received only two intravitreal methotrexate injections (400 ug/0.1 mL each) OU prior to entering hospice care.

KEY POINTS

- Vitreoretinal lymphoma is a rare, intraocular malignancy that can present in all layers of the posterior segment. In particular, the vitreous, retina, and subretinal pigment epithelial space are affected.
- Histologically, primary VRL is an aggressive form of diffuse large B-cell lymphoma.
- About 90% of patients will develop central nervous system (CNS) involvement, although unilateral, isolated VRL may have decreased risk for developing CNS disease.
- Currently, there are no adequate treatment protocols. Initiating systemic and local therapy in eyes with isolated VRL may decrease CNS involvement but not decrease all-cause mortality.
- First-line local therapy includes intravitreal methotrexate first line or rituximab second line in populations that are CD20 positive. There are various protocols for administration, but typical treatment course is for 1 year.
    - Example treatment protocol for intravitreal methotrexate:
        - 4 injections, once weekly
        - 4 injections, biweekly
        - 9 injections, monthly
        - Total treatment course = 12 months

CHAPTER 66

Retina Combined Hamartoma

Eric D. Hansen ▓ Elizabeth L. Turner ▓ Brandon Kennedy

Decreased Vision in a 14-Year-Old Female

HISTORY OF PRESENT ILLNESS

- A 14-year-old female presents with decreased vision over the past year in the left eye. She recently lost her eyeglasses, and her optometrist noted diminished best corrected visual acuity on repeat refraction. The patient acknowledges blurry vision that has gotten gradually worse. She has no previous ocular history or trauma. No family history of ocular pathology or retinal disease other than refractive error.

Exam

	OD	OS
Visual acuity	20/30	20/100
IOP (mm Hg)	17	17
Sclera/conjunctiva	Quiet	Quiet
Cornea	Clear	Clear
AC	Deep/quiet	Deep/quiet
Iris	Normal	Normal
Lens	Lamellar cataract	Lamellar cataract
Anterior vitreous	Clear	Clear
Retina/optic nerve	Normal	Peripapillary, minimally elevated lesion involving retina and RPE with overlying gliosis, variable pigmentation, macular striae, green-gray juxtafoveal lesion concerning for CNVM (Fig. 66.1)

AC, Anterior chamber; *CNVM,* choroidal neovascular membrane; *IOP,* intraocular pressure; *RPE,* retinal pigment epithelium.

QUESTIONS TO ASK

- Has your child shown any signs of decreased vision in the affected eye(s)?
- Does your child have any other relevant medical or ocular history?
- Questions about NF1/NF2 neurocutaneous syndrome
  - Is there any history of neural tumors in the family?
  - Has your child ever shown signs of hearing loss or vertigo?
  - Does your child have a history of seizures?
  - Does your child have any skin nodules or hyperpigmentation?

No financial interest associated with the manuscript. No funding supports.

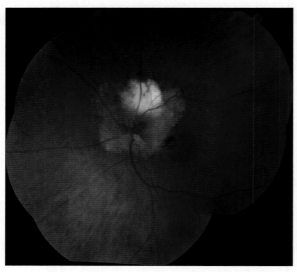

Fig. 66.1   Peripapillary CHRRPE with well-demarcated borders at the level of retinal pigment epithelium, variable pigmentation, and overlying gliosis at vitreoretinal interface.

The child complained of blurred vision for 1 year. She has no family history of benign or malignant tumors and has no other relevant medical history.

ASSESSMENT

- Peripapillary lesion involving the retina with retinal pigment epithelium (RPE) changes, pigmentation, and preretinal gliosis
- Gray juxtafoveal lesion concerning for choroidal neovascular membrane (CNVM), OS
- Bilateral lamellar cataracts

DIFFERENTIAL DIAGNOSIS

- Choroidal melanoma (adults)
- Retinoblastoma (children)
- Congenital hypertrophy of the retinal pigment epithelium (CHRPE)
- Congenital simple hamartoma of the retinal pigment epithelium (CSHRPE)
- Astrocytic hamartoma
- Epithelioma (adenoma) of the RPE
- Toxocariasis
- Morning glory phenomenon
- Choroidal nevus

WORKING DIAGNOSIS

- Combined hamartoma of the retina and retinal pigment epithelium, retina combined hamartoma (CHRRPE), OS

INVESTIGATION AND TESTING

- Optical coherence tomography (OCT) showed peripapillary lesion with full-thickness retinal involvement, disorganization of retinal architecture, loss of ellipsoid zone layer, and irregularity of RPE (Fig. 66.2A). Preretinal membrane formation with sawtooth appearance and a fibrovascular pigment epithelial detachment (PED) with overlying intraretinal fluid are also present (Fig. 66.2B).
- B-scan ultrasound of OS showed hyperechoic elevated peripapillary lesion with no evidence of calcium and medium-high, irregular reflectivity.
- Fundus autofluorescence of peripapillary CHRRPE showed hypoautofluorescence secondary to RPE involvement of the lesion (Fig. 66.3A).
- Fluorescein angiogram (FA) of OS showed tortuous intralesional vessels with areas of hyper- and hypofluorescence in early phases of angiogram corresponding to RPE changes and hyperpigmentation (Fig. 66.3B). Later phases of FA demonstrated hyperfluorescence of peripapillary tumor and juxtafoveal leakage corresponding to presumed CNVM.
- Genetic testing for *NF2* was negative.

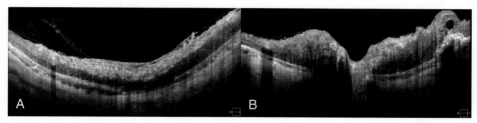

Fig. 66.2 Ocular coherence tomography images of combined hamartoma of the retina and the retinal pigment epithelium (CHRRPE) demonstrating (A) full-thickness retinal involvement with disorganization of retinal layers, preretinal fibrosis, and involvement of RPE/basement membrane (BM) and (B) choroidal neovascular membrane with intraretinal fluid complicating peripapillary CHRRPE. Note the mini sawtooth appearance of the inner retina in the image.

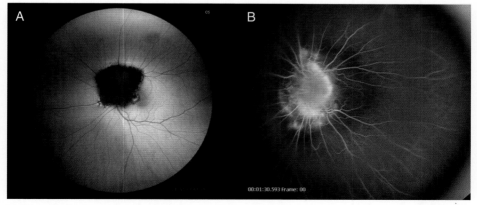

Fig. 66.3 (A) Fundus autofluorescence of peripapillary combined hamartoma of the retina and the retinal pigment epithelium with hypoautofluorescence secondary to retinal pigment epithelium involvement of the lesion. (B) Fluorescein angiography in midphase revealing vascular tortuosity and hyperfluorescence due to leakage.

MANAGEMENT

- Patient underwent exam under anesthesia with intravitreal anti-VEGF therapy for secondary CNVM.
- No indication for vitreoretinal surgery; recommend observation of early preretinal membrane formation.
- Referral to pediatric ophthalmology for amblyopia management and monitoring of mild lamellar cataracts.
- Educate the patient and/or family about visual prognosis and the potential for secondary complications such as CNVM, macular traction, and exudation.

FOLLOW-UP

- Repeat exam in 1 month and imaging following anti-VEGF.

KEY POINTS

- CHRRPE are rare, presumed congenital tumors thought to arise from glial cells of the inner retinal layers. Eventually, they often progress to further retinal and RPE involvement.
- Common CHRRPE tumor characteristics include slight elevation, varying degrees of pigmentation, contraction of the inner surface due to vascular tortuosity, and distortion of normal retinal architecture. They most often are located peripapillary, extending in fanlike projection, but they can also arise extramacular.
- CHRRPE have a known association with neurofibromatosis type 2 (NF2)—an autosomal dominant congenital neurocutaneous syndrome that affects organs of ectoderm origin, especially the skin, central nervous system, and eyes. Patients with NF2 can present with bilateral CHRRPE involvement. Reports of association with NF1 and other congenital disorders have also been made.
- There is no curative management for CHRRPE—rather, therapy is commonly aimed at the preservation of visual quality. Conservative care options generally involve observation and amblyopia management. More aggressive interventions involve anti-VEGF therapy in the presence of CNVM or PPV with membrane peeling in cases of adherent vitreous and/or significant epiretinal membrane (ERM) formation. Additionally, patients should be educated about signs and symptoms of a worsening condition.
- Although CHRRPE is a benign lesion, it commonly causes visual disability. The prognosis for these patients generally depends on tumor location, size, and amount of retinal traction; vision loss can be expected over time.
- Possible complications include retinal exudation, retinal detachment, and vitreous hemorrhage.

Note: Page numbers followed by "*f*" indicate figures, "*t*" indicate tables.